COVER UP
The Facts They Don't Want You to Know

Nicholas Hildyard

KU-318-464

NEW ENGLISH LIBRARY

To my nieces Henrietta and Alexandra, in the hope that they will grow up in a world which has learnt to live without cover-ups.

First published in Great Britain in 1981 by
New English Library Ltd

Copyright © 1981 by Nicholas Hildyard
Copyright © 1983 revised and updated paperback edition
by Nicholas Hildyard

First NEL Paperback Edition revised and updated August 1983

NEL Books are published by
New English Library,
Mill Road, Dunton Green,
Sevenoaks, Kent.
Editorial office: 47 Bedford Square, London WC1B 3DP

Typeset by Fleet Graphics, Enfield, Middlesex

Made and printed in Great Britain by Cox & Wyman, Reading

British Library C.I.P.

Hildyard, Nicholas
    Cover up.
    1. Pollution
    I. Title
    363.7'32   TD174

    ISBN 0-450-05562-0

CONTENTS

I would like to thank the many people who gave so generously of their time and knowledge to help me research this book. In particular, I am indebted to: Bob Alvarez, Hilary Bacon, Dr Irwin Bross, Barry Castleman, Brian Cope, Dr Samuel Epstein, Jim Garrison, Dr Thomas Mancuso, Dr Andrew Marino, Dr Thomas Najarian, Danny Sheehan, Dr Alice Stewart, Dr Joseph Wagoner, Dr Charles Wakstein, Eleanor Walters and Karen Wilson. I would also like to thank those at The Environmental Policy Institute, The Christic Institute, Aruppe House, the Citizens Hearings on Radiation Victims, The Atomic Veterans Association and The Library of Congress.

I would like to express my gratitude to Carina Cooper, Ruth Lumley-Smith, Camilla Bayne-Powell, David Boisseau, Dale Thurstan, Jennifer Heymann, Marjorie Naisbitt, Maria Parsons, Mandy Rickard, Sarah Coombes, Betty Gibson, Meriel Salt, Charles Carey, Rupert Birley, Kathy Goldsmith and the numerous others who gave so much help and encouragement.

Finally, I owe special thanks to Edward Goldsmith for his unstinting support and inspiration, to Peter Bunyard, to Victoria and James Anderson, to Ginnie Clotworthy and Hilary Datchens for undertaking all the typing, to Nicholas Dale-Harris and Belinda Kirkin for editing the manuscripts, to my parents, to Michael and Caroline Salt for not only lending me their cottage but also for their kindness and generosity whilst I wrote the hardback edition of the book, and above all, I owe special thanks to Anne Goldsmith.

Withiel, 1983

COVERING UP THE FUTURE

IN OCTOBER 1980, Mr Trevor Brown, head of the chemical division at Aldermaston responsible for processing weapons-grade plutonium, was officially reprimanded by the Ministry of Defence. His offence was a statement on a BBC television programme that 'an obsession with secrecy had possibly lowered safety standards (at Aldermaston)'.

Clearly, such a statement cannot be construed as jeopardising our national defence. Nor can Mr Brown be accused of untruthfulness; indeed his thesis has now been vindicated at an official inquiry conducted by Sir Edward Pochin.

What he was in fact accused of is: failure to cooperate with his employers in covering up the now established fact that employees at the nuclear establishment are being subjected, during the course of their work, to unacceptably high levels of radiation.

The only object of such a cover-up is to permit the perpetuation of conditions that must ultimately condemn a lot of people to a slow and lingering death from cancer or to the psychological torture of bringing up malformed children. This, most reasonable people would concede, is a more anti-social thing to do than to, say, rob a bank and thereby simply deprive a few people of their surplus cash. Yet unlike a bank robbery it is, in effect at least, quite legal.

The law provides no means of preventing the government and industry from concealing information from the public, nor from providing it with misleading or indeed downright false information, which Mr Brown would undoubtedly have been expected to do had he been Aldermaston's spokesman on safety matters.

What Mr Brown has been reprimanded for is, in fact, nothing more than his refusal to join a callous and cynical conspiracy to commit what should unquestionably be regarded as a serious crime.

If this incident were an isolated one there would be no need for Nicholas Hildyard's book, but of course it is not. In the last decades, the public has been misinformed and indeed deliberately lied to, over and over again, both by industry and government to render acceptable to it activities which may be desirable on short-term and political and economic grounds, but *which are highly undesirable on biological, ecological and social grounds and hence totally contrary to the medium – and long-term interests of the public.*

What is more, many of these activities, I am quite sure, would never have been accepted by the public if their true effects had not been so systematically and unscrupulously dissimulated. This is undoubtedly the case with the spraying of 93 per cent of our crops with synthetic organic pesticides, residues of which are present in just about all the food for sale in our shops.

It is undoubtedly the case with the re-treatment of spent fuel at Windscale which is leading to the irreversible contamination of the Irish Sea and of its fish life with caesium and plutonium, and it is also the case with the purposeful contamination of our food by the food-processing industry with known carcinogens such as the coal-based artificial colourants.

The trouble is that if the public does not rapidly become aware of the extent to which it is being misinformed on such critical matters then the economy will have become so totally dependent on the continuation of these highly polluting activities that they will have become virtually unstoppable. For instance, once our industry has become totally dependent for its electricity on nuclear power, even if that dependence is seen to coincide with an escalating cancer-rate, an increase in the number and seriousness of accidents at nuclear installations and a corresponding increase of radioactivity in our environment, the government will have no choice but to continue to deny any correlation.

It is difficult to avoid wondering how the government is going to render acceptable to the public such biologically suicidal enterprises as the projected construction and operation of a range of 1,000-megawatt breeder reactors, or the large scale 'domestication' of microorganisms by means of genetic engineering which must inevitably lead to the exposure of human populations to man-made viruses and bacteria of which they have had no evolutionary experience.

In order to succeed in doing so, cover-up techniques will have to be considerably refined. The cover-up will have to become a fine art – the literary genre of the last decades of the 20th century as the novel was of the 19th and the epic poem of the Homeric Age. It will have to develop a machinery and expertise of its own. It will also need to acquire the sort of funds to pay for the armies of researchers, copywriters and sundry other propagandists. Only then will it be remotely possible to render acceptable to the long-suffering public the Frankenstein-like monsters that our scientists have conjured up, in what can only be a futile attempt to regild their tarnished image and to resuscitate our collapsing economy.

This being so, we must pay a great deal of attention to Nicholas Hildyard's book – and it must inspire a concerted action on the part of all responsible people to prevent the otherwise inevitable development of a 'cover-up society'.

Edward Goldsmith

INTRODUCTION

IN 1973, the British Medical journal *Lancet* carried an editorial warning of a 'a sinister complex of big industrial manufacturing firms' which was deliberately suppressing information about the dangers of many of the chemicals to which the public is daily exposed. 'The medical men and scientists employed by these firms are chiefly concerned with their employers' and their own profits and are indifferent to the health of exposed workers,' the *Lancet* alleged. 'Some of the firms' employers have . . . even ignored legal regulations and got away with it. Another . . . tack is for a firm singly or in combination with like firms to set up supposedly independent research institutes whose scientists seem always to find evidence to support the stance taken by the firm, despite massive contrary evidence. Thus, when some high-sounding institute states that a compound is harmless or a process free of risk, it is wise to know whence the institute or the scientists who work there obtain their financial support. But there are government agents . . . to enforce safety measures and to draw up others, to see that regulations are in force and to monitor dangerous processes. Alas, it seems that these people are too often involved in the medical/industrial complex and are reluctant to enforce regulations, to emphasise risks to employees or to see that measures are taken to warn or protect them against industrial hazards.'[1]

Since 1973, numerous incidents have confirmed the *Lancet*'s allegations. Moreover, it has become clear that the chemical and pharmaceutical industries are not the only culprits. The nuclear industry, the toxic waste disposal industry, the microwave and electricity industries are all tarred with the same brush – and the cover-up mentality appears to be increasingly widespread. In the United States alone, over three-quarters of all indictments brought against companies are for wilfully breaking anti-pollution laws or for flouting health and safety at work regulations, and the number of cases is rising each year as the present recession jades the ecological conscience of our industrialists. 'You will find in more cases than you wish to imagine that the very highest corporate leaders of our nation have consciously decided to conceal a workplace hazard or market an unsafe product because they valued profit over people,' comments George Miller, a congressman from California who recently introduced a bill proposing criminal penalties for those found guilty of covering up health hazards. 'And I think that kind of conduct is a crime,' he added. [2]

Indeed it is: and it is a crime for which no gaol sentence or fine can adequately compensate. For unlike political scandals, the fallout from industrial cover-ups goes far beyond tarnished reputations (which, if Richard Nixon's current popularity is anything to go by, can easily be restored). At issue are thousands of highly toxic poisons – from drugs that can cause birth defects to cancer-causing chemicals and radioactive wastes affecting not only man but the very physical environment on which life itself depends. Indeed, theirs is a legacy which will be paid out to our children and grandchildren not in cash but in increased rates of birth defects, brain damage, cancer and ecological degradation. Are we really prepared to inflict such destruction on subsequent generations? Is it not time that those who callously disregard the health of the public in order to make a quick profit were brought to book?

1
THE DEATH OF
KAREN SILKWOOD

IN 1975, the Nuclear Regulatory Commission, the watchdog of the nuclear industry in the United States, commissioned Professor John Barton to write a report on nuclear power's implications for civil liberties. Barton's report[1] makes it clear that he is concerned at the lengths to which civil authorities may have to go in order to prevent terrorists obtaining bomb-grade plutonium, thus creating a nuclear 'incident'. Even so, Barton appears to take it for granted that special powers will have to be invoked; that lie detectors will have to be used to screen employees at nuclear plants; that wiretapping will have to be sanctioned: that searches of suspects' houses will be necessary whether or not warrants have been obtained; and finally, that torture may have to be used to force terrorists into admitting where they have hidden any stolen plutonium.[2]

Barton's report – leaked in early 1977 – seemed to confirm the anti-nuclear movement's worst fears: the more so, at a time when information was gradually coming to light about the mysterious death of a young laboratory analyst working for the Kerr-McGee Corporation, one of the powerful energy conglomerates in the United States. Owning half the uranium reserves in America, and with numerous oil wells to its name, it is hardly surprising that Kerr-McGee – with annual sales of $2.1 billion and profits at $116 million – should be judged by the prestigious *Fortune* magazine to be the twentieth 'best investment' in the country.[3] More surprising, however, are the conditions at the company's nuclear installations – and the circumstances surrounding the death of one worker who tried to improve them.

Shortly after seven o'clock on the evening of 13 November 1974, Karen

Silkwood left a downtown café in Crescent, Oklahoma, and headed south along Highway 74. It had been a fraught day, spent negotiating a new union contract with her employers at the Kerr-McGee (KM) Nuclear Facility in Cimarron, just a few miles outside Crescent. Now, after a two-hour debriefing session, she was on her way to a meeting in Oklahoma City. On the seat beside her lay a thin manilla folder, allegedly containing proof that KM officials were deliberately falsifying vital safety tests at the plant. That file, Karen told a friend as she left the café, would 'get Kerr-McGee once and for all.'[4]

Forty miles away, an investigative reporter for the *New York Times* waited patiently for Karen to arrive. She never did. Just outside Crescent, her car sped off the road, skidded for a hundred yards, slewed into a ditch and smashed into a concrete culvert, killing her instantly. Before the night was out, Kerr-McGee officials had rummaged through the wreckage. The manilla folder was never seen again. And later, an independent investigator would testify that, in his opinion, Karen's Honda Civic had been hit from behind by another car moments before she crashed. Just how, and why, was Karen Silkwood killed?

Brought up in Nederland, Texas, Karen knew all too well the meaning of pollution.[5] On a still day, the smog from the local oil refineries hangs in a thick pall over the town. One can literally taste the oil in the air. For Karen, nuclear power spelt an end to that gagging stench. Bent on a career in science, she won a scholarship to college and elected to read chemistry and physics. She never completed the course, however, for she soon fell head over heels in love and dropped out after a year to get married. Seven years later, her marriage on the rocks, she upped sticks and abandoned Texas for Oklahoma. Hearing that Kerr-McGee's Nuclear Division was hiring laboratory assistants to work at its Cimarron plutonium plant, she eagerly applied for the job.

The Cimarron facility had been built in 1970 after Kerr-McGee was awarded a $7.2 million contract to manufacture fuel rods for an experimental 'fast' breeder reactor designed by Westinghouse. Next door was another plant turning enriched uranium into pellets to fuel the country's light water reactors. By the time Karen arrived, both facilities had an unenviable reputation for accidents, sloppy workmanship and numerous contamination incidents.[6]

Two years after her death, Professor Karl Z. Morgan, one-time director of Health Physics at the prestigious Oak Ridge National Laboratory, told a committee of the United States Congress that he had 'never known an operation in the nuclear industry that was so poorly run from the standpoint of radiation protection'.[7] Among other things, Morgan charged that employees were inadequately trained and that many of them seemed unaware of the dangers of the materials they were handling. Indeed, some did not even know that plutonium causes cancer. In one incident, a young teenager brought a popgun to work and fired uranium dioxide fuel pellets at his colleagues whenever he got bored.[8] Others used the pellets as paper weights or threw them around the main production room as a game. One worker allegedly took a pellet of uranium home to give to his son to take to school, and others used to 'race' each other to see who could get contaminated the fastest. In the uranium plant, the uranium dust was so thick that it covered the floor – but no one seemed unduly concerned. As one worker put it: 'What did I care so long as it didn't stain my shoes?'

'The place was a pigpen,' says Jim Smith, a former supervisor at Cimarron. 'The plant was so thoroughly contaminated that to make the building safe, you'd have to break it up and put the whole thing in a nuclear burial ground.'[9] Contamination incidents were legion. Pipes leaked, spilling plutonium solution on to the floor, sometimes a foot deep. The rubber gloves used to handle the plutonium fuel pellets often had holes in them. To save time, safety precautions were deliberately flouted. Rather than clean up a 'hot' room immediately, workers would be given respirators – often for a week or more – until they found the time to break off production and clean up the area. Frequently, the respirators didn't fit and many workers preferred not to wear them, particularly on minor tasks. Indeed, one employee reports that when the rubber gloves in the metal glove boxes where the fuel rods were assembled needed replacing, it was common to turn the glove boxes away from the radiation monitors and perform the change-over without protection. Even when hot wastes had to be scooped from the glove boxes, some workers would carry out the job without respirators, placing a guard outside the room to make certain that no prying supervisors were about.[10]

Kerr-McGee's management seemed oblivious to the dangers of such practices. They were oil men at heart, brought up in the hard world of wildcat oil strikes, blowouts and massive spills. 'They were used to cleaning up 50,000 barrels of oil in two days,' Jim Smith told a BBC *Panorama* reporter. 'They couldn't understand that if you spilt just one teaspoonful of plutonium, you put the plant out of commission for two to three weeks. They just couldn't believe it.'[11]

Smith, who had worked for twenty years in the nuclear industry, recalls one occasion when a room became so 'hot' that, even after a cleaning-up crew had repeatedly scrubbed the walls, the place was still 'screaming'. Kerr-McGee officials simply sent Smith to a local discount store, told him to buy a hundred gallons of whitewash and set him to paint the walls. It took nineteen coats to cover all the flecks of plutonium that couldn't be washed off. The ploy worked for a day or so, then the paint began to flake off in thick sticky chunks, recontaminating the room and everyone in it. The room was never properly decontaminated.[12]

In another incident, two maintenance workers were splashed with plutonium when they were fixing a pump. Their contamination wasn't discovered until they returned from lunch at a café a few miles from Cimarron. They had plutonium in their hair, on their hands and faces; even their car was contaminated. Yet Kerr-McGee never sent a team to monitor the radiation levels at the café where the men had eaten. And in open violation of the government's guidelines, they failed to notify the US Atomic Energy Commission of the incident.[13]

Karen was incensed at the conditions at the plant and, after working there just three months, she joined a strike to protest against the appalling health and safety standards. For ten weeks, she and her colleagues in the Oil, Chemical and Atomic Workers Union (OCAW) bravely held out against Kerr-McGee. But the company remained adamant that there would be no compromises. As if to drive home the point, untrained 'scab' labour was brought in to keep the production line rolling. Contamination incidents continued apace. By early spring, the strikers' will had been sapped and, in dribs and drabs, those who had not lost their jobs to scab labour drifted back to work. To add insult to injury, KM demanded that they sign a new contract, stripping them of their privileges and offering fewer protections against arbitrary dismissals. For the union, it was a dismal, demoralising defeat.

Three weeks later, a bag of plutonium waste burst spontaneously into flames, spewing radioactive dust into the air and contaminating seven workers. The company doctor, who lived an hour's *flying* time away from the plant, was not notified until the following day. When he arrived, it was found that the company had run out of the special chemicals needed to decontaminate the workers. Four days later, the seven men still hadn't been given a full medical check-up, and it took more than a week before faecal samples (the best indicator of the extent of internal contamination) were taken. It was estimated that the workers had inhaled 400 times the permitted weekly intake of plutonium. In fact, no one knows how badly the men were really contaminated for the air monitors in the room were 'out of order' on the day of the fire. [14]

This time, however, the incident did not go unrecorded. For Karen was, by now, taking scrupulous notes on every accident at the plant and every infringement of AEC guidelines. After the humiliation of the strike, she was determined that the next battle with Kerr-McGee would be fought on ground of her choosing. She knew that a dossier of well-documented health and safety violations would prove a weapon powerful enough to bring even the mighty Kerr-McGee Corporation to its knees. And she intended to use it.

Having broken the OCAW strike, KM went gunning for the union. In the early part of 1974, the company began a well-orchestrated campaign to strip OCAW officials of their mandate to represent Cimarron workers in their pay negotiations. The issue was to be put to the vote in early October, just a month before a new pay deal was scheduled to be negotiated. As things stood in the summer of 1974, the union knew it had little chance of winning the vital vote; worse still, Karen and her colleagues realised that their defeat would remove the one force protecting workers at the plant. The time had clearly come to play the union's trump card: Karen's dossier on health and safety violations at Cimarron.

On 27 September, Karen Silkwood – by now a full-time OCAW officer – flew to Washington. With her were Jack Tice, president of the local branch of OCAW, and his colleague, Gerald Brewer. The three of them met with officials of the Atomic Energy Commission and testified, behind closed doors, that Kerr-McGee was violating numerous safety standards. Among other things, they charged that KM had failed to keep radiation levels as low as practically possible; that in some cases the company had ignored radiation standards altogether; and that KM had failed to educate their workers adequately about the dangers of plutonium. Altogether, Karen and her colleagues lodged 39 specific complaints, 20 of which were later substantiated.[15]

The AEC officials duly took note of OCAW's allegations but stressed that they could do nothing without documentary evidence to back up the charges. In the meantime, they said, they would continue to make regular 'spot' checks on the Cimarron plant to see if OCAW's charges could be substantiated. In fact, the AEC never made a single 'spot' check during the whole five years that the plant operated. Every time AEC officials were due to visit Cimarron, the plant's director of health and safety, Wayne Norwood, was telephoned by a contact at the AEC and told exactly when the 'surprise' inspection would take place *at least a week* in advance. During that week, former workers allege, production would be halted, whole areas cordoned off and decontaminated, and the plant thoroughly cleaned up.[16]

Whilst in Washington, Karen casually mentioned to Antony Mazzochi, the national president of OCAW, that she had evidence that Kerr-McGee officials were falsifying safety tests on the fuel rods being manufactured at the plant. The eight-foot long rods, filled with plutonium pellets, are sealed at both ends with welds that must be free of any flaw if they are to operate safely. No one knows for certain what would happen if, once in position, the rods were to leak and release radioactive gases; it is thought, however, that the flow of liquid sodium used to cool the core of a fast breeder reactor could be interrupted, causing the rods to overheat and, possibly, leading to a meltdown. Karen alleged that X-rays of faulty rods were being 'doctored' by laboratory technicians using a black magic marker to paint out any hairline cracks that showed up on the negatives.[17]

'They were the most serious charges I have ever heard in my career as a union officer,' recalls Mazzochi.[18] After that afternoon's meeting with the AEC, it was clear, however, that Karen's allegations would be dismissed out of hand by the authorities unless she could provide firm evidence to support them. That evening, Mazzochi and his assistant, Steve Wodka, took Karen to one side: could she obtain copies of the doctored X-Rays? The batch numbers of the faulty rods that had been passed as safe? The names of those falsifying the negatives? And, above all, the names of Kerr-McGee officials who knew the tests were being rigged?

For the next month, Karen devoted herself to collecting the material needed to substantiate her charges. On the pretext of working late, she stayed on at the plant after her shift ended, pouring over files she had surreptitiously obtained from KM's executive offices, photocopying incriminating documents and noting every safety violation. On 7 October, she telephoned Wodka in Washington to tell him that faulty welds were still being passed, 'no matter what they look like, no matter what the pictures look like.'[19] She went on to report that she had got hold of one weld that had been ground down so far in an attempt to smooth out scratches and imperfections that it had to be discarded.

Three days after that telephone conversation, two professors from the University of Minnesota came to Cimmaron to talk to plant workers about the dangers of plutonium. Both men were well versed in their subject: Dr Dean Abrahamson was a medical doctor and a nuclear physicist; and Dr Donald Geesaman had been a top AEC scientist for thirteen years, but had been sacked after campaigning for stricter radiation exposure standards. The two professors were horrified when they heard of the frequency and nature of past contamination incidents at Cimarron. Since the plant opened, they were told, 73 workers had been exposed to airborne plutonium. Karen had been one of those contaminated and she was visibly shocked when Abrahamson told his audience that the chances of those who inhaled plutonium contracting cancer within the next fifteen to thirty years was 'disturbingly high'. Surely, she asked, she would be safe if the amount of plutonium she had inhaled was below the exposure limits set by the AEC? Not so, said Abrahamson: if plutonium could be measured in the air, the levels were already too high; moreover, the AEC guidlines were the subject of a heated debate within the scientific community, with some experts claiming they were meaningless.[20]

After the meeting, Karen gave Abrahamson and Geesaman a lift to the airport. On the way, she asked them what she could do about conditions at the plant. Their advice was unequivocal: if she valued her health, she ought to find another job. But Karen didn't. She continued to work undercover and by the end of October she had what she wanted: a copy of a doctored X-ray and the name of the laboratory assistant who had painted out the telltale cracks. She telephoned Wodka with the news on 2 November. He was delighted, telling Silkwood that he would contact David Burnham, an investigative reporter for the *New York Times*, and fly with him to Oklahoma City on 13 November so that Karen could hand over the documents in person. Burnham would then write up the story during the week of the vital pay negotiations, embarrassing Kerr-McGee and strengthening OCAW's bargaining position. In the meantime, Wodka advised, Karen should lie low and take things easy.

What he didn't realise, however, was that by this time Kerr-McGee knew all about Karen's activities – and had done for the past fortnight. Already Karen was in deep trouble.

On the night of 12 October, Karen dined with her boyfriend, Drew Stevens, at a pizza restaurant just outside Crescent.[21] Halfway through dinner, she noticed three young men snooping around her car. Thinking they might be part of a gang which had stolen her cassette tape recorder a week earlier, she asked Drew to investigate. Frightened that there might be violence, Karen also called over the restaurant's security officer, an off-duty policeman called Bill Byler. Drew and Byler checked out the youths, found nothing suspicious and returned to the restaurant.

Over a cup of coffee, Karen complained to Byler about conditions at the Cimarron plant, spelling out the dangers of plutonium and railing against Kerr-McGee's constant safety infringements. Byler was clearly interested in what Karen had to say, and when a friend of his, Steve Cambell, joined their table, Karen suggested that they all went over to her apartment to continue the conversation as the pizza house was about to close.

Almost the first thing that Byler saw when he walked into Karen's flat was a hooker and other paraphernalia normally used for smoking marijuana. He didn't say anything – he was off duty, after all – but the evidence that Karen took drugs clearly preyed on his mind. As the evening wore on, the conversation turned to fast cars and then to hunting. At this point, Byler asked Karen if she had any guns. No, she replied, she hadn't; adding jokingly, 'But Drew's got a couple of M16 automatic rifles in the back of his car.' Drew explained that his roommate Bob Ivans, was a marksman in the National Guard and withdrew the guns each weekend for target practice. 'I just happened to have borrowed his car this evening,' Drew told Byler. 'If you want to see them, you're welcome.' The two men left the apartment, looked at the guns securely locked in the boot of Ivan's car, and returned upstairs for another drink.

That chance meeting probably sealed Karen's fate. The next morning Byler went straight to Bob Hicks, commander of the Special Intelligence Unit of the Oklahoma City Police Department (OCPD). When Hicks heard Byler's report of events the previous evening, he ordered an immediate investigation of Karen and her associates. Strangely, it never occurred to anyone at the OCPD to telephone the National Guard and establish that the M16s had indeed been legally withdrawn from the National Guard's armoury by Ivans. Instead, Hicks set up a meeting with Jim Reading, chief of security at Cimarron and Hicks's former boss at the OCPD. Convinced that Karen was a threat to Kerr-McGee's security, Reading suggested that the Intelligence Unit slap a wiretap on Karen's telephone. Even though it is illegal under Oklahoma law to conduct electronic surveillance without a special federal court order, Hicks readily agreed with Reading's plan. From that moment, Reading (who was in constant contact with Hicks) knew Karen's every move.

On 5 November, Karen went to work on the afternoon shift, leaving the laboratory, where she was testing various samples of plutonium, at about 5.30 p.m. for a tea-break. On the way out, she went through a routine check for skin contamination. The needle on the radiation monitor went crazy, registering plutonium levels forty times higher than those deemed safe by the AEC.[22] Karen was rushed for emergency decontamination, stripped, scrubbed with wire brushes and sent home early. Meanwhile, Kerr-McGee laboratory workers inspected the glove box where Karen had been working: there were no signs of any radiation leak, nor was the room, itself, 'hot'. The source of Karen's contamination remained a total mystery.

The next day, Karen returned to work. Again the radiation monitor went crazy; again she was put through the painful process of decontamination; and again the source of her contamination couldn't be traced. This time, however, a nasal smear showed that her contamination was internal and Karen was ordered to report the next day to the Health Physics Department to have her sinuses drained in an attempt to prevent the plutonium reaching her lungs. By now, Karen was hysterical. In desperation, she rang Dr Abrahamson to ask his advice. 'She knew what the medical implications were,' Abrahamson later told Howard Kohn of *Rolling Stone* magazine, 'and she was worried.'[23]

She had good reason to be. Five years later, Dr John Gofman would testify before a federal jury that, in his opinion, Karen was 'married to cancer' as a result of her contamination. Gofman, the scientist who first invented the process for isolating plutonium, was at pains to point out the awesome power of plutonium to cause biological damage. Plutonium, he explained, is a highly unstable element and as it decays, it emits 'alpha particles', charged nuclei of helium which travel at thousands of miles per second. 16 grains of plutonium, each weighing one-billionth of a gram, emit 2,000 alpha particles every second, he told the court. And each of those particles delivers 5 million volts of energy – two and a half million times the amount of energy obtained from burning a lump of coal. To expect a cell to survive being hit by an alpha particle without suffering any biological damage, he said, is like expecting a delicate Swiss watch to work perfectly after someone had taken off its back and rammed an ice-pick through it. 'It's such an absurd notion that one wonders how anybody can think of it.'[24]

On the morning of 7 November, Karen reported to the Health Physics Department for the sinus-draining operation. Yet again she was found to be contaminated: her hands, face and arms showed high levels of plutonium; a faecal sample she had brought with her registered 30,000 disintegrations per minute (sixty times higher than the AEC ceiling); and a nasal smear registered 45,000 dpm.[25] Karen broke down. It was the third time in three days that she had been found to be contaminated. Worse still, it was now clear that the source of her contamination was not within the plant. That left only one other place: her home.

Sherri Ellis, Karen's room-mate, was asleep when Kerr-McGee officials, dressed in protective 'moon suits', arrived to check the apartment for plutonium contamination. The air-conditioning system was dismantled, desks and chests of drawers were emptied, curtains were ripped down, carpets torn up and pots, pans, towels and sheets were seized and put into a 55-gallon drum for burial at one of Kerr-McGee's nuclear waste tips.

It soon became clear, however, that the KM inspection team was looking for much more than the source of Karen's contamination. During the search, Karen's diary (together with other personal papers) was impounded and handed over to Jim Reading – even though it showed no signs of radioactivity. Silkwood's private monthly budget book was also reviewed and seized, presumably because it contained an entry for marijuana. Reading and his colleagues from Kerr-McGee's security division emptied the medicine cupboard in the bathroom, taking away a bottle of pills that Karen had on prescription, a beaker and a syringe. A bag of marijuana found in the living room was also seized. 'It was a full scale search,' recalls Jim Smith, the plant supervisor, alleging that Reading was really looking for any evidence which could be used to discredit Karen as an OCAW negotiator.[26]

Indeed, it was not until the next day, 8 November, that AEC inspectors were called to the scene. Only then was the source of Karen's contamination discovered: when the inspectors opened her refrigerator, their geiger counters screamed. The bologna and cheese which Karen had been eating registered 400,000 disintegrations per minute.[27] The flat was immediately sealed off and all the remaining furniture removed.

Meanwhile, Karen, Sherri Ellis and Drew Stevens had all been sent to a government radiation laboratory in New Mexico for full medical check-ups, which included internal examinations and whole-body scans. Hearing the news, Wodka assumed that the planned meeting with Burnham would have to be called off.[28] But four days later, Karen telephoned him from Los Alamos: Kerr-McGee had failed to find the vital documents during their raid on her apartment as she had hidden them elsewhere.[29] She knew they were safe, she said, and that night she would fly back to Oklahoma, make a surprise appearance at the union negotiations the next day, and then drive to Oklahoma City to meet with Burnham. She had already arranged for Drew Stevens, by now discharged from hospital, to pick the reporter up from the airport.

The next evening, Burnham, Wodka and Stevens sat in a room at a Holiday Inn waiting for Karen to arrive. The minutes ticked by. Eight-thirty. Nine o'clock. Nine-fifteen. By now Wodka was worried: Karen was over an hour late. He tried to telephone her to find out what had gone wrong but, for some mysterious reason, the hotel's telephone system was temporarily out of order. It was not until 9.45 that he managed to contact Jack Tice, president of the local branch of OCAW. Half an hour later Tice rang back: Karen was dead.

The three men sped off in Burnham's car towards Crescent. They arrived at the scene of the accident to find that Karen's car had already been towed away and that her body had been taken to the local morgue.

Wodka immediately suspected foul play, and at crack of dawn the next morning, after a fraught night identifying Karen's body and trying to locate her car, he went to the offices of the local Highway Patrol. There he was told that the police were treating the accident as a classic case of 'falling asleep at the wheel'.

Wodka was far from satisfied; the more so when he and Drew Stevens finally found Karen's car at a local garage and learned that Kerr-McGee officials had searched the car during the night. According to Ted Seabring, the owner of the garage and the man who had towed away Karen's car, a radio operator from the Highway Patrol had telephoned him shortly after midnight and told him to allow the KM men complete access to the car.[30] Although Seabring cannot recall any documents being removed, he does remember the Kerr-McGee officials reading aloud a letter to Karen from a friend in Canada. What is certain, however, is that Trooper Rick Fagen, the first police-man on the scene of the accident, saw a bundle of papers with Kerr-McGee's distinctive letterhead in Karen's car before it was towed away. Indeed, he later testified that he had made an agreement with Roy King, an executive at Kerr-McGee, to meet and remove the papers, but found that it wasn't necessary, for by the next morning, 'somebody else had already done the job'.[31]

In any event, by the time Wodka and Stevens arrived at Seabring's garage, the papers were nowhere to be found. Apart from $8 in cash, all that remained of Karen's personal effects were two marijuana 'joints', a Mickey Mouse wristwatch, an identity card, a small note-book, and an electronic security key.[32]

Three days after the accident, A.O. Pipkin, an ex-policeman and an expert in reconstructing accidents, arrived in Crescent at the request of Wodka. He examined Karen's car and the site of the crash, taking numerous photographs and measurements. He was left with several nagging questions which needed answers before he could rule out any possibility of foul play. Why, for instance, had Karen swerved left *across* the road before crashing? If she had fallen asleep, wasn't it more likely that she would have veered to the right, hitting the culvert on the side of the road on which she was driving? What, too, about the skid marks on the left-hand verge of the road? Their pattern indicated that Karen's car had been out of control before it even left the road; yet the police had ignored them in their report. And how had the two fresh dents in the rear bumper of Karen's car been made? During the crash? When the car was towed away? Or by another car?[33] Pipkin's conclusion was unequivocal: 'There is enough circumstantial evidence present to indicate that the car was struck from behind by an unknown vehicle, causing it to go out of control, due to the initial impact or the combined impact and driver overreaction.'[34]

The local Highway Patrol were adamant, however, that Karen had fallen asleep at the wheel. And, if she hadn't, they argued, she had crashed because she was on drugs. Certainly, Karen had been taking 'quaaludes', sleeping pills which had been prescribed by her doctor, for several weeks before her death – and an autopsy had found 0.35 milligrams of methaquaalude in her bloodstream. But would this small amount be sufficient to send her to sleep after only five minutes at the wheel? Yes, said Dr A.J. Chapman, who had performed the autopsy on Karen. No, said eight independent pharmaceutical experts: medical reports, they pointed out, showed that Karen had been taking two quaaludes a day for three months prior to her death and had probably developed a high tolerance for the drug. Under such circumstances, it was highly unlikely that the pills would have impaired her driving ability.[35]

When Tony Mazzochi, Wodka's boss at OCAW, read Pipkin's report, he immediately filed a formal complaint with the US Department of Justice, calling for a full investigation into the circumstances surrounding Karen's contamination and death. Whether or not her death had been accidental, any investigation would clearly cause embarrassment to both Kerr-McGee and those involved in her surveillance and harassment.

FBI agent, Larry Olson, was assigned to the Silkwood case a week after Karen's death. A confidential Kerr-McGee memorandum from Jim Reading to Dean McGee, chairman of the board, makes it clear that, from the outset, the thrust of Olson's investigation was to uncover 'the means used by *Silkwood* to remove plutonium from the Cimarron facility'.[36] Olson, who had developed a hand-in-glove relationship with Kerr-McGee (and Jim Reading, in particular), was convinced that Karen had contaminated herself in order to embarrass the company.

At first, he played with the fanciful story that Karen had removed plutonium from the plant by smuggling it out up her vagina and had then contaminated her apartment on returning home. His explanation for the high levels of radioactivity in Karen's refrigerator was still more perverse: 'The AEC had no idea how it got there,' he told Howard Kohn, 'and I didn't either. For a while I thought she might have been abusing herself with a ring of baloney and that the plutonium had gotten on that way. But I checked and found that it was sliced baloney'.[37]

If he had checked further, he would also have found that the plutonium which contaminated Karen came from a batch which was locked in a vault to which she had no possible access.[38] He didn't, however, and in March 1975, he closed his investigations. His final report accepts at face value the theory of the Oklahoma State Patrol, that Karen had fallen asleep at the wheel, and dismisses outright OCAW's allegation that documents Karen was carrying had been removed by Kerr-McGee officials. Indeed, Olson maintained that such documents could never have existed, since Kerr-McGee executives had assured him that Karen's charges were untrue – and therefore impossible to document. Finally, Olson reported that it was impossible to determine exactly how Karen's apartment had come to be contaminated.

But whilst Olson was still convinced that Karen was to blame for her contamination, he had drastically altered his views on *why* she was contaminated. It seemed probable, he now argued, that Karen would contaminate herself to embarrass the company; after all, there had been so many previous contamination incidents that one more was unlikely to cause a major stir. Instead, Olson had come up with a new – and extremely alarming – theory.

According to Howard Kohn, the *Rolling Stone* journalist who broke the story, Olson learnt through press reports in 1975, that Kerr-McGee was having problems with its plutonium inventory. National Public Radio charged that 40 pounds were missing and David Burnham of the *New York Times* put the figure as high as 60 pounds – worth some $10 million on the black market.[39] In fact, when the plant was closed in 1976, 22 pounds were unaccounted for. The company claimed that the plutonium was still stuck in the plant's pipes and simply needed to be flushed out. But Jim Smith, the plant's supervisor, told Kohn: 'We could have flushed for another month and we wouldn't have gotten another three ounces out of that sonofabitch.'[40] So where had the missing plutonium gone?

'Olson's curiosity was aroused,' reports Kohn. 'Silkwood had been contaminated with plutonium; that was indisputable. The plutonium had come from the Kerr-McGee plant; that was a near certainty. Some 40-60 pounds of plutonium were unaccounted for; that appeared to be a well-grounded allegation. Olson developed a theory: Silkwood had been stealing plutonium.'[41]

Olson persuaded Ted Rosack, his immediate superior at the FBI's Oklahoma office, to support a request to headquarters in Washington for permission to investigate further the 'Silkwood smuggling ring'. Without explanation, Washington turned down the request; Rosack was posted to Denver; and Olson was firmly told that the case was considered *closed*.

There the matter might have rested, had it not been for the determined efforts of Kitty Tucker, legal coordinator of the Washington DC chapter of the National Organisation of Woman (NOW). Tucker first heard of Silkwood when she read a report in the *Washington Post* which gave prominence to Kerr-McGee's claim that Karen had contaminated herself.

'I knew the charge was ridiculous,' recalls Tucker, who persuaded NOW to take up the cudgels on behalf of Silkwood and OCAW. In

August 1975, Tucker, together with Karen DeCrow, president of NOW, and Sarah Nelson, NOW's labour coordinator, led a delegation to the Justice Department to protest against the constant delays in the official investigation into Karen's death. They were told that, as far as the Justice Department was concerned, the Silkwood case was closed and that if they expected the FBI to solve every case, they must 'have been watching too much television'.[42] The three women were dumbfounded; not even Karen's parents had been informed that the case was closed. And when they asked that the Justice Department make its findings public, they were told that it was official FBI policy not to discuss 'closed' cases.

'The Justice Department had closed the investigation without filing a single charge,' Sarah Nelson told newsmen after the meeting. 'Plutonium couldn't just grow in her refrigerator. Someone had to put it there.'[43]

Tucker and her colleagues were undeterred by the Justice Department's cries of 'No case to answer'. Through NOW, they launched a national campaign to lobby for Congressional hearings in the Silkwood affair. Members of NOW, other civil rights groups and environmental organisations all showered Senator Abraham Ribicoff, chairman of the powerful Senate Committee on Government Operations, with letters demanding an investigation, not only into Karen's death, but also the FBI's handling of the case. On 18 November 1975, Ribicoff agreed to hold hearings and assigned the task of organising them to Senator Lee Metcalf, a Democrat from Montana.

But they had underestimated Kerr-McGee's reach. Two weeks before the hearings were due to begin, Dean McGee flew in from Okhlahoma City for a secret meeting with Metcalf. The next day, Metcalf announced that the hearings were to be cancelled and issued a press statement claiming that Silkwood's parents and OCAW were satisfied with the Oklahoma Highway Patrol's original explanation of Karen's death. Silkwood's parents and the union vigorously denied Metcalf's claim.[44]

Win Turner, general council to Metcalf's committee, and Peter Stockton, the Senate investigator who had been assigned to help prepare the case for the committee, were totally taken aback by Metcalf's announcement. Their initial investigations had already led them to believe that there was far more to the Silkwood case than the Justice Department and the FBI were prepared to admit. Off their own bat, they had found out about the forty pounds of missing plutonium, yet Stockton was expressly denied permission to interview Olson and officials from the Nuclear Regulatory Commission (which had taken over from the AEC as the watchdog of the nuclear industry) about the missing plutonium. William Brock, a member of the Senate Committee on Government Operations, told him that Kerr-McGee's plutonium inventory was none of his business and that he was overstepping his authority in trying to investigate it. [45]

Out of the blue, Stockton was then approached by a young woman journalist, Jacque Srouji, who urged him to call off the Senate investigation. Srouji claimed that Karen Silkwood was mentally unstable, a mother who had callously deserted her children, a drug addict and a frustrated divorcee. Any attempt to make a heroine out of her would only serve to embarrass Congress and should be avoided at all costs. But the crunch came when Srouji announced that she could back up all her allegations with documentary evidence: to prove her point, she produced copies of a number of typescripts of telephone conversations made by Silkwood which she admitted had been 'bugged' by Jim Reading and Bob Hicks. [46]

Stockton was amazed. If the FBI were practising illegal wiretapping and electronic surveillance, it was no surprise they did not wish their involvement in the case to be made public. Indeed, when he tried to obtain Olson's file on the case, the Justice Department refused to part with it, claiming that it had an official policy never to discuss 'closed' cases. [47] When it was pointed out that 'closed' files had, in the past, been handed over to Congress, the FBI declared that the Silkwood case had been 'reopened due to all the inquiries being directed to the bureau'. In the event, Stockton did manage to obtain a heavily edited copy of Olson's file: but conspicuously missing from it were the letters Olson had sent to headquarters explaining his theory of a smuggling ring at Cimarron.

In spite of this obstruction and Metcalf's cancellation of the scheduled hearings, Stockton determined to pursue the case. He quickly persuaded Congressman John Dingle, a Michigan Democrat who chaired the House of Representatives' Sub-Committee on Energy and the Environment, to reopen the hearing. Almost immediately Dingle was flooded with protests from Kerr-McGee and the FBI, who both argued that his committee would be breaking its official brief if it stepped into the Silkwood affair. The committee's funds were cut off. An official complaint was filed by Tom Stead, the Congressman from the district of Oklahoma City where Kerr-McGee has its headquarters. And, later, Stockton was to receive a mysterious telephone call from a stranger who pleaded for the hearings to cease. 'The FBI will never tell you the truth,' he said. 'They can't afford to. Just forget the whole thing. Give it up. You're in over your head. This thing is so complicated you'll never figure it out. You'll just go crazy trying.'[48]

Despite the pressure on him to call off the hearings a second time, Dingle soldiered on, and, in late April 1976, the hearings opened. Jacque Srouji was one of the first witnesses. Again, just as she had in her private conversation with Stockton, she tried to discredit Karen's character. During the course of researching a book on nuclear power, she said she had interviewed 'numerous associates of Karen who indicated – through official and documented evidence – that she used marijuana and had attempted suicide on at least two occasions, both attributed to drug overdoses'.[49] She then went on to suggest that OCAW might have arranged Karen's contamination in order to create a martyr. However, she claimed, the dents in the rear of Karen's car had been caused when Karen drove off the road some two weeks before her death in order to miss a cow, adding that, at the time, Karen was 'increasingly dependent on quaaludes'.

Under cross-examination Srouji was asked how she had obtained the documentation which she claimed supported her allegations. Her reply created pandemonium. An FBI agent involved in the investigation, she calmly admitted, had given her access to all the confidential FBI papers relating to the Silkwood case, even allowing her to photocopy them. Dingle was aghast. Why had a mere journalist been permitted to read FBI files which the bureau had steadfastly refused to release to the Congress of the United States? Clearly, Srouji's connection with the US intelligence service was closer than she cared to acknowledge.

Michael Ward, the laywer appointed to Dingle's committee, immediately telephoned Larry Olson. The FBI agent, whom Srouji hadn't named, denied that he had ever given anyone outside the bureau access to the Silkwood file and remained tight-lipped. 'Srouji,' he said curtly, before slamming down the telephone, 'has a special relationship with the FBI which I am not at liberty to discuss.'[50] In fact, it later transpired that Srouji was no less than a paid FBI informant, working directly with Larry Olson, and that she also had ties with the CIA.[51]

No sooner was this information out than FBI agents were sent to find Srouji in an attempt to get her to sign a sworn statement that she had *never* received any official FBI documents. This, despite an earlier sworn statement (taken during what Srouji described as a 'grilling' immediately after her appearance at the Dingle hearings[52]) giving a detailed account of how she had obtained access to the Silkwood file, but admitting that she 'had never *officially* received documents from the bureau'.

The Senate committee never had the opportunity to re-examine Srouji, however, for the hearings were not to reconvene after the traditional autumn recess. John Dingle returned to his home state to campaign for re-election to the Senate, only to be accused of being a client of a call-girl who had close contacts with the Mafia. Later, it emerged that the call-girl had been urged to make the accusation by her roommate, a fellow prostitute and an informant for the FBI.[53] Although Dingle was re-elected, the damage had already been done: he was stripped of his position as chairman of the House Sub-Committee on Energy and the Environment – at the express demand of Tom Stead, the Congressman from Oklahoma City – and the second session of hearings into the Silkwood case were declared 'cancelled'.

Once again, the investigation into Karen's death had been halted before it had even really got under way. And, once again, the most powerful authorities in the United States seemed responsible.

One of those present at the Dingle hearings was a young lawyer, Daniel Sheehan, who was acting as a legal adviser to NOW in the Silkwood case. Sheehan is something of a maverick and his career at the Bar has been meteoric. Not only has he worked for some of the most prestigious legal firms in the United States, but the cases in which he has acted as legal counsel read like a roll call of civil rights milestones: the Black Panther bombing conspiracy, the Daniel Elsberg spy trial, the Attica Prison riots, the Pentagon Papers case and the Serpico investigation into police corruption in New York City.

In the autumn of 1976, Sheehan was approached by Karen Silkwood's parents and asked to file a civil suit against Kerr-McGee for damages to their daughter. Now that Dingle had been jockeyed from his position as chairman of the House Committee on Energy and the Environment, they explained sadly, a civil suit appeared the only course open to them if justice was to be won for Karen. Sheehan offered his services free of charge, but asked to be able to examine the evidence further before making any commitment to file a lawsuit.

By early November 1976, Sheehan was satisfied that there was indeed a case for Kerr-McGee to answer, and on 8 November – just five days before the standard two-year statute of limitations on civil lawsuits came into force – he filed a three-count lawsuit alleging that Kerr-McGee was liable for Silkwood contamination; that Kerr-McGee officials, together with agents of the FBI, had participated in a wilful conspiracy to violate the civil rights of Silkwood by illegally 'bugging' her apartment; and, finally, that those involved in the conspiracy had attempted to 'cover up' their activities.[54]

Whilst investigating the Silkwood case, Sheehan began to ask himself just what it was that the FBI seemed so intent on covering up. As a young trial lawyer, he had made many useful contacts amongst the nation's top private investigators – and it was to two of his old friends in this fraternity that he now turned. When they had heard the background to the Silkwood case, both men volunteered their services free.

With Kerr-McGee's surveillance of Silkwood uppermost in their minds, they began to look for similar cases of harassment by the nuclear industry of its critics. In the early summer of 1977, they got the lead they were looking for: a tip from a source in the intelligence community told them that they would find 'all they wanted to know in Georgia'.[55] So, to Georgia they went. There they began looking into the activities of the public relations division of the Georgia Power Company and, in particular, its 'Risk Management Section', run by a Mr Arthur Benson. His immediate colleagues were two men named Bill Lovin and John Taylor, under whom were a dozen or so other employees – all of whom had been former intelligence officers for either state or federal police forces. It soon emerged that Benson and Lovin were running an office involved in more than public relations: they were part of a national network of private security companies organised to conduct illegal surveillance of anti-nuclear activists and other 'dissident' groups.

Lovin showed the Silkwood investigators the files kept by Risk Management on 'dissidents'. Each was neatly catalogued under headings such as 'sexual difficulties', 'financial problems', 'civil liberty activity' and 'anti-nuclear sympathies'. Within the files, there were reports on local dignitaries, anti-nuclear activists, the local director of the American Civil Liberties Union, and workers at a nearby nuclear plant.

Inquiries within the intelligence community revealed that Lovin, Taylor and Benson had all spent a considerable time before organising Risk Management at the National Intelligence Academy, a shadowy private school specialising in clandestine political surveillance. Subsequent investigations also revealed that the NIA ran a company which sold wiretapping equipment. The company, Audio Intelligence Devices, had supplied the very wiretaps that were used to bug Karen Silkwood.

'The picture was bizarre, but it was beginning to fit together,' recalls Sheehan. 'In August 1977, the Silkwood investigators obtained the name of a woman who had served as the private secretary of Captain Bill Vetter, the commander of the Intelligence Unit of the Oklahoma Police Department. In interviews with this woman, it was learned that in 1971 Vetter had used federal law enforcement assistance administration grants, given to the State of Oklahoma by the US Justice Department, to purchase wiretapping equipment, electronic eavesdropping equipment and long-range photographic surveillance equipment to be used by the newly created Intelligence Unit within the Oklahoma City Police Department. The woman also confirmed that Bill Vetter had been engaged, throughout the entire period of her employment by the Oklahoma Police Department's Intelligence Unit, in illegal wiretapping, breaking and entering and electronic surveillance. She said that she had personally typed the typescripts of wiretaps. The wiretaps had apparently been carried out by the Intelligence Unit's officers "in their unofficial capacity". Their targets included the Black Muslims; members of the radical Students for a

Democractic Society; Abby Hoffman, the anti-Vietnam war campaigner; and Iranian students suspected of smuggling arms.'[56]

Whilst the links between the Oklahoma City Police Department, Audio Intelligence Devices and Georgia Power's Risk Management were all being pieced together, Sheehan established that shortly before her death, inquiries had been made by another nuclear power company about Karen Silkwood. The inquiry came through a Sacramento-based organisation called the Law Enforcement Intelligence Unit. According to one policeman, who worked undercover for the group, 'The LEIU is so secret that until recently even its existence was denied'.[57] Effectively a private club of police officers, its overt purpose is to circulate and computerise information on organised crime. Something of the flavour of the LEIU's activities can be gleaned, however, from a report by investigative journalist George O'Toole: 'One undercover officer who infiltrated a Chicago group and eventually became its president . . . admitted before a grand jury probing police spying activities that he had specifically urged other members of the organisation to shoot Chicago policemen and had even demonstrated the most strategic way to place snipers in downtown Chicago so that they could blow away the greatest number of his fellow officers.'[58] And, whilst the LEIU claim to have no truck with the surveillance of political activists, Sheehan claims to have evidence that information about Silkwood and her activities was entered into the LEIU computer.

On 6 March 1979, the lawsuit brought by Karen's parents came to court before Frank J. Theis, an out-of-state judge who had been asked to preside over the trial after the impartiality of two Oklahoma State judges, Luther Eubanks and Luther Bohanan, had been called into question. Six months earlier, Eubanks, who had originally been appointed the trial judge, described the Silkwood's case as 'not worth a row of beans' and accused Sheehan of 'running off at both ends'.[59] The Silkwood lawyers immediately filed a motion to have Eubanks removed from the bench but, before the motion came to court, Eubanks (who had apparently been tipped off) handed over the case to his colleague, Luther Bohanan.

Bohanan was less outspoken in his remarks but, nonetheless, his bias was pronounced. Nominated by Kerr for the job in 1961,

Bohanan had always maintained a close friendship with the Senator. Indeed, when Bohanan's nomination was turned down by President Kennedy on the grounds that he was 'unqualified', Kerr flexed all his political muscles and stubbornly supported the appointment in the face of widespread opposition. When a journalist asked him who his three choices were for the job, he is reported to have said: 'Bohanan, Bohanan, Bohanan.' In the event, Kerr got his way and Bohanan was duly appointed district judge for Oklahoma City. [60]

Bohanan was eventually removed from the bench after the Silkwood lawyers won an appeal to have the case heard by an out-of-state judge and, in February 1978, Theis was appointed as judge. The day the trial opened, Theis told the crowded courtroom; 'There are a lot of ghosts in this case and I'm either going to bury them once and for all, or they're going to get up and walk.' [61]

On 18 May 1979, the jury awarded $10.5 million to the Silkwood estate. Earlier, Theis had established a legal precedent by ruling that US nuclear power companies could be held liable for any health damage to the general public from low-level radiation – a decision which has major implications for the nuclear industry, particularly in the wake of near-meltdown at the Harrisburg nuclear plant in March 1979. In effect, the ruling opens the doors for a flood of compensation claims from workers and members of the public injured by radiation – and the defence that they assumed a risk by, for example, living near a nuclear plant will no longer be valid.

Two other charges against Kerr-McGee and various FBI and Oklahoma police officers – alleging a conspiracy to deprive Silkwood of her civil liberties and an attempt to cover up the circumstances surrounding her death – have still to come to court. Whether the mystery of Karen's death will be resolved remains to be seen. Did she indeed fall asleep at the wheel of her car? Or was she murdered? And if so, why? To retrieve the documents in the missing folder? Because she knew too much about the illegal wiretaps on her home? Because she had stumbled across a smuggling ring? No one will ever know for certain but, whatever the final verdict, Karen will remain a potent symbol of the civil liberties that may be lost if we embrace a nuclear future. As one group of anti-nuclear activists daubed across a Kerr-McGee poster advertising the benefits of nuclear power: 'Ask Karen Silkwood . . . She should know'.

2
DOWN IN THE DUMPS

WITHIN THIRTY years the seas will be dead. That prediction was made throughout the early seventies by Commander Jacques Cousteau, and his concern is shared by many of the world's top marine biologists. For years, industry has used the seas as a convenient dump for its most dangerous toxic wastes – and the results have been disastrous. Every year Britain, alone, dumps some 124,000 tons of mixed industrial and domestic wastes into the Irish Sea; 29,000 tons into the Bristol Channel; 288,000 tons into the North Sea; and 86,000 tons into the English Channel.[1] By 1979, those waters received 23.5 million tonnes of waste from Britain.[2] The practice has wrought ecological havoc, but it is a cheap solution to a pressing problem and, consequently, government and industry alike have played down its environmental dangers.[3]

Many of the chemicals dumped have 'sublethal' effects we are only just beginning to understand: they don't kill outright, but lead to genetic damage, behavioural defects, disorientation, fin lesions, reduced fertility and an inability to reproduce.[4] Either way, they can result in the disappearance of entire marine species – threatening our food supplies and, ultimately, the ecological balance on which our own survival depends. And for every pollution incident we know about, there are ten more which have been successfully hidden from the public.

One of the worst offenders is undoubtedly the nuclear industry.[5] The Windscale nuclear reprocessing plant, for example, discharges 136,000 curies a year of radioactive caesium directly into the Irish Sea, and it is now well documented that these and other radionuclides are building up in the sediment of the seabed at a rate much faster than their annual rate of disintegration.[6] Studies by the Ministry of Agriculture, Fisheries and Food also show a steady movement of radioactive material from Windscale northwards round the tip of Scotland and into the northern North sea. So, too, plutonium released into the sea from France's reprocessing plant at La Hague on the Normandy coast has migrated up the Channel and is now found in high quantities on the north coast of Germany.[7] Nobody knows for certain the ultimate fate of these radioactive wastes or their effects on marine life, but the contamination is already widespread.[8]

In America, the problem of toxic waste is particularly acute. Major fish kills in the Mississippi have now been traced to the tons of pesticides washed off the surrounding farmlands. Oysters caught off Long Island Sound, New York, show alarmingly high levels of cadmium,[9] a heavy metal which can lead to high blood pressure and (in the worst cases) to irreversible kidney damage, a breakdown in the body's ability to replace bone tissue and, ultimately, to a total collapse of the skeleton.'[10]

In the Mediterranean, pollution is growing daily. Quite apart from the vast quantities of oil discharged illegally from ships, some 430,000 million tons of pollutants are dumped into the sea each year via the rivers of Europe – 360,000 of phosphorous; 21,000 tons of zinc; 2,400 tons of chromium, and untold quantities of raw sewage. The Rhône, alone, releases into the Mediterranean some 30,000 tons of oil, 700 tons of phenols, 1,250 tons of detergents and 500 tons of pesticides. Indeed, mussels caught near the French-Italian border contain up to 4,000 parts per billion of DDT, and fish in the area have three times the maximum level of mercury considered safe for human consumption.[11]

Just occasionally, the terrifying effects of such indiscriminate dumping are brought home to the public. In the summer of 1953, for instance, villagers in the fishing town of Minemata, Japan, noticed their cats staggering around the harbour.[12] By December, doctors were reporting a dramatic increase in the number of children and adults suffering convulsions, blindness and a lack of co-ordination.[13] Within the next eight years, 43 people in Minemata died of this strange disease and a further 68 were permanently disabled from cerebral palsy.[14] The cause: mercury discharged into Minemata Bay in the industrial waste from a nearby chemical plant owned by the Chisso

Corporation.[15] For years, the company denied responsibility for the disaster.[16]

America, too, has suffered its own dumping tragedy. In December 1975, all fishing was banned in the James River, Virginia, after the US Environmental Protection Agency (EPA) discovered high levels of the pesticide kepone in fish and mud samples.[17] The company responsible for the contamination, Life Science Products of Hopewell, had discharged the pesticide into the local sewage system with the full knowledge of Hopewell's city council.[18] The kepone-contaminated sewage sludge flowed directly into a tributary of the James River and ultimately into Chesapeake Bay. Moreover, the sludge was virtually untreated since the kepone had interfered with the natural breakdown of the sewage and, indeed, contaminated the whole sewage treatment plant, rendering it inoperable. Although the municipal authorities knew of this problem, they neither alerted the State Water Pollution Control Board nor the EPA for seven months.[19] Fish from 'as far away as the Atlantic Ocean off New Jersey' were found to be contaminated.[20] In 1981, the ban on commercial fishing in the James River was lifted. This despite evidence that fish in the river were still contaminated with kepone at levels above those considered safe for human consumption.[21]

Nor is the problem confined to the pollution of our rivers and seas. Billions of tons of hazardous industrial wastes have been indiscriminately dumped down isolated mineshafts, into local streams, into poorly run landfills and onto derelict land. These toxic Gomorrahs are now beginning to take their revenge. In the United States alone, it will cost some $6 billion to prevent them from exacting untold ecological damage and a further $40 billion to ensure that they are rendered harmless.[22] Indeed, many US officials privately confess that the problem is now beyond control and that it is only a matter of time before the toxic timebomb beneath America explodes. Meanwhile, the public is being kept in the dark as to the true extent of the danger.

Evidence is steadily mounting that the present methods of disposal – in the main, landfill – are far from satisfactory. Even more alarming, it appears that industry (particularly in the United States but, increasingly in Britain also) is turning to illegal dumping in an attempt to get rid of its wastes. If that trend continues, then widespread contamination of the environment is not just a possibility: it is inevitable.

The reaction of government has been predictable: toxic waste legislation has, invariably, proved the Cinderella of the statute books, continually delayed or watered down – usually at the behest of industry. In the USA, controls on toxic waste disposal have been dramatically relaxed by the Reagan administration.[23] Meanwhile, Britain's Department of the Environment has reduced the number of 'notifiable' wastes by two-thirds and instituted new controls which have been described as 'unworkable, inadequate and virtually unenforceable.'[24] Government, it would seem, is now a willing partner in the attempt to suppress or play down the dangers of toxic waste dumps. Concern for profitability of industry has won the day – and the inevitable loser will be the general public.

For years, the residents of Love Canal, a quiet suburb of Niagara City and a stone's throw from the US-Canadian border, complained of noxious fumes in their basements, fumes that they believed originated from a disused toxic waste dump beneath their housing estate. For its part, the local health authority showed little interest in the problem and still less desire to investigate. In the summer of 1978, however, the residents' worst fears were realised. The prolonged and heavy snows of the previous winter had caused water to seep into the dump site, causing it to overflow and forcing the chemicals out into the soil. A thick black slime began to appear on the surface, covering gardens and oozing into basements. An immediate inquiry was ordered and three months later, Governor Carey of New York State announced that all 235 families would have to be evacuated. Shortly afterwards, President Carter declared Love Canal a federal disaster area, the first ever instance of a national emergency being caused by chemical pollution. Still more families had to be moved when it was discovered that the toxic waste was migrating further afield via underground streams.

'I used to have quite a few friends who lived up there,' a young man, just out of the army, told me. 'But the authorities moved them out after the disaster and I haven't been able to trace them since. It's sad when man pollutes himself out of house and home.'

We were talking in a bar some two miles north of Love Canal. An hour before, I had taken a taxi to visit the abandoned housing estate. Driving out from Niagara City, we passed a three-mile stretch of chemical plants: Dupont, Hooker Chemicals, Allied Chemicals, Ascension Chemicals . . . factory after factory, separated only by scrubland littered with broken-down cars and discarded, rusting drums. Like so many people in this highly industrial city, the taxi driver had his own stock of pollution stories.

'The office where I work daytimes is just a few blocks from here,' he told me. 'The air's so bad that the paint in my room has turned black and keeps flaking from the walls. If those chemicals do that to paint, imagine what they must be doing to my lungs! Myself, I live near a disused waste dump and they've found just about everything down there – from dioxin to that pesticide which killed so many fish in Lake Erie. Mind you, it's not as bad as the place we're going to: that's the bottom line in disasters.'

It was snowing heavily by the time we reached Love Canal and the drifts were beginning to build up against the eight-foot high fence that now surrounds the old estate. Large notices warn that the area is contaminated and out of bounds to those without special permits. Inside the perimeter fence, I could see the abandoned houses, their doors and windows boarded up. Even so, the looters had clearly had a heyday. In one garage, its doors ripped off their hinges, a chest of drawers lay smashed to pieces, its contents strewn across the floor along with the remains of a child's bicycle whose tyres had rotted away from its wheels. As for the house behind the garage, it was now no more than a shell, burned out by arsonists.

'We've had quite a few looters up here,' said the taxi driver. 'Some of the families didn't take their furniture with them when they moved, so the pickings were there for the taking. But the people I feel really sorry for are those just across the street from the Canal estate. They're still living there. They can't sell their houses. They haven't received a cent in compensation. And do you know why? Because the authorities say this road marks the limit of contamination.'

Love Canal takes it name from William T. Love, a nineteenth-century entrepreneur who planned to build a model city near Niagara Falls. Part of his ambitious scheme involved digging a seven-mile canal which would connect the upper and lower levels of the Niagara River in order to exploit the falls for cheap hydroelectricity. Work on the canal began in the summer of 1895 but, before it could be completed, economic recession put paid to Love's dream, his backers deserted him and the project was abandoned.

In the early twenties, the partially dug section of the canal was bought by the Hooker Chemical Corporation (now a subsidiary of the giant Occidental Petroleum Corporation) and used as a dump for toxic wastes. Almost 22,000 tons of chemicals were buried there before the site was eventually capped with clay and covered with earth in 1953.[25] Hooker Chemicals then sold the canal to the Niagara Falls Board of Education for one dollar, on condition that the company was absolved of all responsibilities for any injury which might result in the future from the chemicals buried beneath the site.[26] An elementary school was built on the old dump, along with a housing estate and it appears that at some stage during the building programme, the clay cap sealing the dump site was severely damaged. Hence the leaching of the chemicals.

It now appears that Hooker knew about problems at the site as early as 1958, after it was reported that children had been burned by leaking chemicals. An internal memorandum reveals that two Hooker officials inspected the site, which was being used as a playground, and found that 'the ends of some drums . . . were exposed and south of the school there [was] an area where benzene hexachloride spent cake was exposed'.[27] The two officials recommended that the chemicals should be 'recovered' but, although the company claims it notified the Niagara Falls Board of Education about the leaking chemicals, there is no record in the NFSB's files to confirm that it did so.[28] Indeed, the same memorandum explicitly states that it was felt that the company 'shouldn't do anything unless requested to by the school board'.[29]

In August 1978, the extent of the contamination at Love Canal was first made public.[30] An initial study, ordered by Dr Robert Whalen (who was New York State's Commissioner for Health at the time that the crisis first blew up) identified 82 different chemical compounds – 11 of them known or suspected carcinogens.[31] Subsequent investigations revealed 200 other compounds, only half of which were identified. It was estimated that at least 10 per cent of these chemicals would prove carcinogenic, mutagenic or teratogenic.[32]

The Whelan study also revealed that the frequency of miscarriages in the Love Canal area was 1.5 times higher than the expected rate within the general population:[33] miscarriages among those living around the southern end of the Canal were almost 3.5 times the normal rate, as were the number of birth defects.[34] That study (which led to the first evacuation) was followed by another of Dr Beverly Paigen of the Roswell Park Memorial Institute. Chemicals from the Canal, she argued, were migrating along old streams which once criss-crossed the neighbourhood, spreading the contamination far beyond the immediate borders of the Canal. Those living in houses built over the streams – in what Paigen termed 'wet' areas – showed higher rates of 'miscarriages, birth defects, nervous breakdowns, asthma and diseases of the urinary system' than those living in 'dry' areas.[35] Indeed, Paigen found that 1 in 5 children born in 'wet' areas had birth defects, compared with 1 in 14 in 'dry' areas. Moreover, the incidence of birth defects was apparently rising dramatically: between 1974 and 1978, half of the children born in 'wet' areas were deformed.[36] Although New York State's Health Department initially rejected Paigen's findings on birth defects, it eventually decided to recommend the 'temporary' evacuation of pregnant mothers and children under two years of age. Paigen has since alleged that she was harassed after she took up the cause of Love Canal's residents – an allegation described by Whalen's successor, Dr David Axelrod, as 'grossly untrue'.[37]

The controversy over the true extent of the contamination at Love Canal (a controversy which is by no means over) was further fuelled by a 1980 report which claimed to have found rare chromosomal aberrations (involving not only breaks in the DNA chain but also strange additions) in 30 per cent of local residents.[38] Normally such aberrations would be expected in 1 out of every 100 individuals.

The results of that study, commissioned by the EPA and carried out by Dr Dante Picciano, a genetic toxicologist from the Houston-based Biogenics Corporation, were leaked to the *New York Times* the day before they were due to be announced. A spokeman for Hooker Chemicals described the conclusions of the study as 'premature' and argued that they would cause 'unnecessary anxiety' among the residents of Love Canal.[39] Later, a review panel, set up by the Department of Health and Human Services, criticised Picciano's work on methodological grounds.[40] Those criticisms were endorsed by a second review panel, convened this time by the EPA. A third independent panel, however, supported the study.[41]

Today, Love Canal is being recapped with a new layer of clay.

Three other Hooker dumps around Niagara Falls are now known to pose severe health hazards. One of the dumps, at Bloody Run Creek, has been described as 'a waste-pile' which is potentially 'a more serious long-term problem for the environment than even Love Canal.'[42] Hundreds and possibly thousands, of pounds of dioxin – one of the deadliest chemicals known to man – are estimated to have been dumped in the site and significant traces of the chemical have been found in the Niagara River and in Lake Ontario.[43, 44] The dump is just across the road from a water treatment plant serving 100,000 people.[45]

Some $14 billion worth of lawsuits have now been filed against Hooker.[46] Nonetheless, the plight of Love Canal's former residents is by no means over. In 1982, the EPA published the results of an $8 million study on the Canal. It concluded that the chemicals dumped there had not migrated much beyond the houses immediately bordering the old dump site. For reasons that are not entirely clear (some claim a cover-up: others blame bureaucratic bungling) the final recommendations of the report were altered twice shortly before its release. At first, the study team concluded that the area could be reinhabited; then it argued that no recommendation could be made; and finally (just one day before the report was released) it reaffirmed its initial conclusion. Small wonder that two Congressmen, Representatives Alfone D'Amato and John LaFalce, alleged that the final conclusions had been reached because EPA and State officials had 'put the pressure on'.[47, 48]

Whatever the truth of that allegation (it has been rigorously denied), critics point out that the study is in any case badly flawed. According to Nancy Haneson of *New Scientist,* only four samples of soil were taken from Ring 3 (the evacuated area furthest from the Canal); samples of highly volatile chemicals were kept for months before being analysed; and the laboratories where samples were tested 'differed as much as 30-fold in their measurements of identical samples'.[49] Indeed, both a review panel from the Department of Health and Human Services and another from the National Bureau of Standards had been extremely critical of the report even before it was published – although they accepted its overall findings.[50]

For its part, Hooker greeted the report enthusiastically. 'The EPA responsibly handled its report,' said Dr Norman Alpert, Vice

President of Occidental Chemicals, Hooker's parent company. 'Any objective scientific analysis of the EPA report would confirm that there are no significant health risks and that the quality of environment in the Love Canal area is similar to many other areas in the United States.' The EPA report, said Alpert, effectively rebutted the claims of the Attorney-General of New York State that Love Canal was a continuing health hazard: 'We urgently request that the Attorney-General refrain from issuing any more meaningless and inflammatory data. The public should demand that all information in the future regarding any chemical contamination must be based on good science and have been subjected to competent scientific review. The public and all concerned deserves nothing less.'[51] Quite.

Love Canal shocked America. The more so when it was revealed that 300 other sites were immediate health hazards; that between 1,200 and 34,000 other sites were thought likely to cause significant environmental problems at some stage in the not too distant future;[52] and that 90 per cent of America's annual inventory of toxic wastes were being disposed of 'improperly, unsafely and irresponsibly'.[53] Indeed, Representative Albert Gore articulated the fears of many when he warned: 'the threat posed by hazardous wastes may be the environmental sleeping giant of this decade. America has been pock-marked with thousands of cancer cesspools – and EPA is dragging its feet to avoid the magnitude of the threat.'[54]

Gore's remarks were made to a 1978 Congressional committee, held to investigate delays in implementing the 1976 Resource Conservation and Recovery Act (RCRA), a bill intended to regulate the proper disposal of toxic wastes. It would take another four years before the EPA finally issued its 'rules' for hazardous waste disposal under the RCRA. When it did, in July 1982, it was amidst accusations that the Agency had bowed to the wishes of industry and watered down the Act. Under the Reagan administration, it was alleged, the Agency had 'suspended, postponed or revised' controls on toxic waste disposal and, in effect, 'assigned industry the responsibility of policing itself'.[55] Environmentalists are primarily alarmed that the head of the EPA's hazardous waste management programme is the former director of communications for subsidiaries of the Aerojet-General Corporation. In 1981, Aerojet's liquid fuel plant was named by the EPA as one of the 40 most contaminated waste sites in the US: indeed, in 1979, the company had been indicted for dumping 20,000 gallons of toxic waste a day into a local swamp. [56]

One of those who is harshly critical of the EPA's record is Hugh Kaufman, assistant to the director of hazardous waste site programmes. 'It's crazy what's going on,' he told Marjorie Sun of *Science* in 1982. [57] Four years earlier, Kaufman had been a principal witness at the 1978 Congressional hearings. At those hearings, Kaufman accused his superiors in the EPA of intentionally covering up the dangers of many known dumps and of blocking efforts to search for other dumps that might prove to be health hazards. [58]

In particular, he cited the case of Summit National Services, a waste disposal firm from Deerfield, Ohio. [59] In 1976, the Summit site was inspected by the Ohio Office of Land Pollution Control after it was learned that two loads of 'C-56' had been delivered to the plant. 'C-56' is a code name used by a particular chemical company in Michigan for Hexachlorcyclopentadiene (HCP), a compound used in the manufacture of kepone (already discredited, as we have seen, in the James River crisis) and Mirex. Not only did investigators find leaking barrels all over the site but, more important still, they discovered that Summit had no facilities whatsoever for handling 'C-56' and that local water courses had been contaminated. The Office of Land Pollution Control recommended that the local EPA office place an immediate ban on further dumping at the site. That recommendation was ignored.

It was two years before Kaufman's department even heard of the case. He contacted the regional EPA office requesting a new investigation and was told in no uncertain terms to get off its back. 'The local office refused even to visit the facility or to let headquarters staff visit,' he reveals. 'They told us to stay out of the region.' [60] Kaufman also discovered, to his consternation, that the Ohio office had several other far more serious cases of hazardous waste dumps on file, but that it had no intention of investigating them either. Still more disturbing, when Kaufman told his superiors of the incident they too chose to take no action.

Nor is this the only evidence that those at the top of EPA were actively opposed to any thorough investigation of potentially hazardous waste facilities. Shortly after the Summit incident, John Lehman, assistant director of the Division of Hazardous Waste

Management and Kaufman's immediate boss, received a
memorandum from Steffen Plehn, deputy assistant administrator for
Solid Wastes.[61] Attached was a complaint from Conrad Simon,
Director of the Environmental Programmes Division that 'headquarters staff' (a thinly veiled reference to Kaufman and his
colleagues) were bypassing regional offices in their search for
hazardous dumps, thus threatening to 'subvert the whole organisa-
tional structure of EPA'. Simon was angry that researchers from Fred
Hart Associates had appeared in a television interview and spilled the
beans on the extent of America's toxic waste problem. 'We feel that it
is inadvisable for EPA consultants to engage in news media interviews
which concern regional interests without prior approval of the appropriate regional office,' said Simon. 'An uncoordinated approach may
lead to serious complications with regard to the release of either
premature, inappropriate, unwise or erroneous information.' Plehn
reacted as Simon clearly intended him to do. He ordered Lehman to
put 'a hold on all imminent hazard efforts'.[62]

Not long afterwards, all regional administrators were sent a request
for information on waste dumps in their areas which might pose
potential health threats. The brief they were given was a limited one,
however. 'It is recognised that the development of this inventory will
add national visibility to the incidents identified therein because the
inventory will be shared with Congress and will probably be requested
by and made available to the public. Because of this, incidents in the
inventory should be situations for which you have more than circumstantial information, the public (at least locally) is already aware, and
publically accessible information is already on file. It is not expected
that EPA make any effort to "discover" sites for which we do not
currently have information.'[63] Put in less bureaucratic language, EPA
headquarters was telling its regional officers that it only wanted to
know what the public already knew. Any other information was to be
kept firmly under wraps.

That unwillingness to disclose pollution incidents to the public is not
unique to the EPA. Internal memoranda reveal that an Occidental
Petroleum plant in Lathrop, California, for instance, deliberately
misled the local water board about chemical wastes leaking into a
nearby well.[64] The plant was manufacturing the pesticide DBCP,
which was later found to be causing high rates of sterility amongst

workers (see page 116). R. Edson, the plant's chief of environmental engineering, warned repeatedly that the company was violating water quality laws, but advised that it would not be 'wise' to inform the authorities. 'For years we have dumped waste water containing pesticides and other products,' he wrote in a 1977 memorandum. 'Fortunately for the management of this company, no pesticide has yet been detected [in a neighbouring well]. I, personally, would not drink water from [the] well. No outsiders actually know what we are doing and there has been no government pressure on us, so we have held back from trying to find out what to do within the funds we have available. Frankly, I don't believe any of us will become TV personalities answering questions on these contaminants. The next drop of pesticide that percolates to the ground is a management decision which I don't feel we can afford. I believe we have fooled around long enough and have already overpressed our luck.'

A year later, no action had been taken. This time Edson wrote that, in his opinion, the company 'has destroyed the usability of several wells in the area.' He went on to warn: 'If anyone should complain, we would be the party named in an action by the Water Quality Control Board. The basic decision is this: do we correct the situation before we have a problem? Or do we hold off until action is taken against us?'

Edson also admitted that he had deliberately misled the water board about the extent of pollution. His report to the board, he wrote, 'was not exactly accurate, even though the inaccuracy is due to omission rather than outright falsehood. However, I don't think it would be wise to explain the discrepancy to the state at this time.'

But perhaps the best documented case of an EPA cover-up comes from a small hamlet some six miles outside Toone, Tennessee. [65] Late in 1964, the Velsicol Chemical Corporation, a Chicago-based company, began disposing of pesticide wastes in a shallow burial site near the hamlet. As early as 1967, a US government geological survey found evidence of contamination of local aquifers and cautioned against further use of the facility. Despite this, the site was expanded and dumping activities were stepped up until 1972 when the site was closed. In 1978, nearly a quarter of a million 55-gallon drums lie rusting at the landfill, and local wells were discovered to be thoroughly contaminated with at least six suspected carcinogens, including carbon tetrachloride, aldrin, dieldrin, chlordane and benzene.

The concentration of carbon tetrachloride was 2,400 times the maximum daily dose recommended for workers by the National Institute of Occupational Safety and Health (NIOSH). When carbon tetrachloride was discovered in Cincinnati's water supply (at levels 48 times lower than at Toone), the EPA immediately warned against drinking the water without boiling it first. No such warning was given at Toone, nor were residents told that carbon tetrachloride could be absorbed through the skin. Indeed, it was only *after* the Congressional hearings that EPA even got around to 'advising' against the use of local well water for bathing or washing clothes and dishes.[66, 67]

Woodrow and Christine Sterling are one family who have been particularly badly affected by the incident, and it is largely through their efforts that the case has received wide publicity in the States. At first the Sterlings showed a touching faith in the integrity of the authorities. Even after tests on their well water revealed positive evidence of contamination, the family continued to drink from it because of repeated assurances from both Velsicol and local health officials that it was safe to do so. 'We drank the water for months,' Mrs Sterling told the Congressional hearings. 'We did not stop because we were not told to stop.'[68]

About this time, Mr Sterling's sister, who lived next door, became pregnant and she, too, continued to drink the local water. Her baby was born two months premature without a stomach wall so that its intestines hung outside its body. 'I was there at the delivery,' recalls Mrs Sterling. 'I asked the doctor if the chemicals in the water had anything to do with it, but he would not take a stand.' In fact, a casual link between pollution from the well and the baby's birth defects has never been established. After the birth, a Velsicol official visited the Sterlings to assure them (again) that the water was safe to drink. When Mrs Sterling offered him a glass to drink, he refused: 'I might die before I get back to Memphis.'[69]

Official obduracy and a general reluctance to get involved in the case was something that the Sterlings were to encounter time and time again. When, for instance, they asked local EPA officials to give them a breakdown of the known effects of the chemicals found in their well water, they were told that it was impossible to provide firm details 'because there hadn't been enough research'.[70] In another incident, blood samples taken from three families in the area remained frozen because the health authorities couldn't find a laboratory to undertake the appropriate tests'.[71]

Throughout the case, Velsicol claimed that there was no evidence to link the poisoning of the wells with their activities at the dump site. In this, the company was supported (albeit tacitly) by the EPA.[72] Official indifference to the case was such that EPA headquarters only learned of the Sterlings' plight through a report on the front page of the *Washington Post* in July 1979.[73] Hugh Kaufman asked Virginia Thompson, a colleague at EPA, to investigate and she immediately contacted the regional office. The transcript of her telephone call is worth reproducing in full:

VT: We are writing damage reports on hazardous waste management. It has come to our attention that there is well water contamination in Hardeman County, Tennessee, which citizens claim is caused by wastes improperly buried by Velsicol. Are you familiar with this case?

Regional Officer: Yes (Silence)

VT: Has the regional office done any investigations of this claim?

RO: Yes (Silence)

VT: Can you tell me the status of your work there?

RO: No (Silence)

VT: You cannot give me any more information? Have you done water sampling or anything?

RO: No, we have not taken samples and I'm not going to tell you anything more about this. Listen, this is a potential enforcement action and you people up there had better stay out of it. I mean, I'm telling your office to *stay out* of this altogether.[74]

An infuriated Kaufman sent an immediate memo to Steffen Plehn, imploring him to intervene and use his authority to force the local EPA to investigate the site. The memo was forwarded to John Lehman, Kaufman's immediate boss, who replied: 'Based on the information in your memo, the problem is, as you say, "perhaps serious". However, a direct link to the Velsicol hazardous waste disposal site apparently has not been established.'

The case was thus closed and Velsicol's claim effectively given the official stamp of approval. Even when a public outcry forced the company to admit that there might conceivably be a connection between the dump site and the well contamination, it still refused to admit liability and only offered local residents $160 in compensation.[75] In November 1979, Velsicol – no doubt disturbed by the bad press it received during the Congressional hearings – finally relented and offered to buy all the houses whose wells had been poisoned.[76]

Perhaps the last word in this tawdry story of deceit should go to its principal victim, Mrs Sterling. 'I don't have words to express how I feel. I am hurt. I am bewildered. Are our daughters going to have deformed children? Is our son going to have deformed children? We have these questions and we cannot get them answered. I feel that the government officials, that the state officials should have been open and honest with us because I thought that is what government was about.'[77]

Kaufman's evidence undoubtedly delivered a body-blow to the EPA's attempts to cover-up the dangers of toxic waste dumps. The Agency was given a public dressing down and ordered to search its files for a complete list of hazardous dumps. But criticism has clearly failed to reform the EPA: it is still (as it always has been) a creature of industry – and industry has proven an uncompromising master.

Early in 1979, President Carter announced plans to create a superfund – bankrolled by industry – to pay for cleaning up abandoned waste dumps. The move angered industry which believed that chemical companies had been unfairly singled out to bear a disproportionate burden of the clean up costs. To support its case, millions of pages of comments were filed on virtually every clause of the proposed legislation. Those comments were described by an EPA official as 'a minefield': 'If we do not handle them properly, industry will be able to use them to go to court to stop or remove our regulations.' In the event, industry had no need to settle its differences in public: its lobbyists went to work and soon it was announced that the target figure for the amount of money to be raised by the superfund had been cut from $4.2 billion to $1.6 billion. Industry was to contribute $1.3 billion through taxes: the rest was to come from the public purse. This against the estimated $28-55 billion in fact needed to clean up America's existing waste dumps.[78]

Meanwhile, a new problem is emerging. In an attempt to avoid the costs of proper disposal, many firms are turning to organised crime to help them get rid of their wastes. As we shall see, a growing number of companies now find the Mafia's cheap 'alternative' methods of disposal increasingly attractive.

Simple mathematics would suggest that if the United States has a waste problem, Britain has a potential disaster on her hands. Although the US produces nearly ten times as much toxic waste as Britain, she has thirty-six times as much land on which to dump it. By that reckoning, Britain's waste disposal dilemma should be three times as bad.

Not so, says the Department of the Environment. 'In my view we do not have the same problems as in the United States and it is invidious to make a comparison,' Anthony Fagin of the Toxic Waste Division told me. 'Britain has a tradition of legislative control which just doesn't hold for the US. We aren't smug about our record but we are satisfied with it.'[79]

That view, however, is difficult to reconcile with the evidence presented before a 1981 Select Committee of the House of Lords.[80] Despite Britain's 'tradition of legislative control', many local waste disposal authorities (WDAs) 'have no disposal facilities for hazardous waste other than asbestos and most are poorly equipped to manage whatever hazardous arisings they have.'[81] By 1981, seven years after they were obliged by law to draw up plans for disposing of the waste produced in their areas, only 12 of Britain's 165 WDAs had actually done so – and London, the biggest waste producer in the country, had not even started on the plan at the time the Committee reported.[82] There is no legislation to prevent waste being imported into Britain 'even if there are no readily available facilities for its disposal'.[83] Many WDAs are 'understaffed or at full stretch' and most (including the Greater London Council) do not even employ a toxicologist.[84] As for the DOE, it was found to have underestimated the tonnage of 'notifiable' waste disposed of in Britain by 2 million tonnes, and, according to one expert witness, the authorities do not even know 'how much hazardous waste is produced in the UK, who produces it, what it is and what happens to it.'[85]

For its part, the Committee concluded: 'Hazardous waste cannot be trifled with, nor can the attitudes of the public who have to live with it. Yet Government (central and local) and the waste disposal industry have only very recently come to terms with the seriousness of the problems which can be created. Too many people are comforted by the belief that because nothing much has gone wrong so far, nothing is likely to go wrong in the future. Constant vigilance will be needed or that comfortable belief could be rudely shattered.'

Nonetheless, the Committee 'was fairly confident' that Britain had no 'Love Canals' festering in her soils. But can we be so sanguine? There is no evidence whatsoever to suggest that British waste hauliers were any more scrupulous than their American counterparts in their dealing with toxic wastes. Until 1972, and the passing of the Deposit of Poisonous Wastes Act (DPWA) – a bill rushed through Parliament after cyanide drums were found abandoned on several sites in the West Midlands – there were no controls (other than the public health acts) over dump sites; there was little control over site selection; and little or nothing was known about how wastes reacted with the soil, let alone with each other.

Indeed, in 1970, a government Committee (later criticised for 'underestimating the seriousness of the problem') warned that many tip operators 'may be living in what may or may not prove a fool's paradise'. The Committee was referring in particular to those manufacturers who were dumping their wastes in tips owned and managed by themselves – a practice the Committee described as 'satisfactory in the sense that the producer of the waste is still responsible for it after disposal' but 'unsatisfactory because the tip site might not have been chosen with toxic wastes in mind'. Almost half of Britain's industrial waste is disposed of in such 'in-house' sites – yet, until 1981, when the DPWA was replaced by new regulations under the 1974 Control of Pollution Act, manufacturers using their own sites were not required to notify local authorities about what wastes they were dumping. [87]

Despite this – and despite evidence that the sixties and the seventies were the heydays of the 'cowboy' operators – the DOE has no inventory of past dumps (those which, if the American experience is anything to go by, are the one most likely to cause problems) and *no intention of compiling one.* Until such an inventory is compiled talk of Britain having avoided a 'Love Canal' is pure wishful thinking. As Bob Keen, principal lecturer in environmental health at Bristol Polytechnic, puts it: 'The balance of probability is that Britain will be very lucky if it can escape the legacy of its buried dumps'. To which Brian Price, pollution consultant to FOE, added: 'The question is not so much a case of "Will a Love Canal happen here?" but "When and how often?"'[88]

'Drivers at the company I worked for were paid a bonus for dumping wastes illegally, usually about three to four pounds a trip', an informed source recalls. 'The licence for one site was revoked after a fire occurred but drivers still continued to use it, sneaking in after dark. In some areas, local authorities were paid to turn a blind eye and at one site we used to dump chemicals along with sewage which we weren't permitted to do. When I complained, I was told to keep quiet or I might lose my job.'

It was allegations like this that led, in 1964, to the British government setting up a special working party, the Key Committee, to investigate the extent of illegal dumping of toxic wastes in Great Britain. The Committee which reported in 1970, documented numerous cases of pollution through 'the burial of cyanides, pesticides, tar sludges and other wastes'. In one case, a borehole investigation of a gravel pit filled with miscellaneous sludges and oils revealed water with a 'biological oxygen demand' ten times greater than raw sewage. In another, cattle and sheep died after drinking water contaminated by fluoroacetamide, rodenticides and pesticides dumped in a nearby field.[89]

In the ten years since the Key Committee, numerous examples of gross pollution through improper, ill-formed or badly supervised disposal have been reported in the national press. A few cases suffice to make the point:

■In 1970, Purle Bros. (Holdings) was prosecuted for polluting Mackelsfield Canal. Purle told the court that it sent a driver to investigate the possibility of using a disused mineshaft near the canal. The driver had emptied his tanker on the site instead of carrying on to an official tip in Nottingham. Two years later, after cyanide had been found dumped on a children's playground, Lord Greenwood was to tell parliament that he found it 'hard to credit the cynical lack of social responsibility' that Purle Bros. appeared to have shown. According to *New Scientist*, 'a director of the company had offered drivers £20 for each new tipping site they discovered and £1 for every load they dumped'. [90, 91]

■The Forestry Commission dumped drums of the herbicide 2,4,5-T down a mineshaft in Wales. According to the manufacturers' instructions, used cans should be washed out in kerosene, crushed and buried beneath three feet of earth. At the time they were found, local health officials claimed that the drums had been properly sterilised. [92]

■Fines totalling £5,200 were imposed on two West Midland companies for illegally dumping toxic wastes on a derelict building site. In another incident – for which the companies were prosecuted – 65 drums of cyanide were deliberately abandoned on a tip near Wolverhampton after tipping permission had been refused. It was alleged in court that an employee at the site had been bribed to allow the load to be dumped. [93]

■A fire at Nettlesfield Quarry at Beith in Scotland resulted in two substantial discharges of lethal quantities of phenolic wastes and cyanide into a nearby river. Subsequent surveys showed that 3,500 fish had been killed. Two years earlier, a number of cows had died near the site after activated carbon containing cyanide, dumped illegally in the quarry was spread on adjacent fields. [94]

■Two West Midland firms, Brasway Ltd. and Brasway Waste Disposal, were charged with conspiring to deposit 'poisonous, noxious or polluting' waste – including cyanide – at three sites in the area. At one site, near Darlaston, 56 tons of cyanide were dumped on to a municipal tip disguised as rubbish. Although the companies had handled cyanide on numerous occasions, they never once notified the local authorities as required by law. The companies were also charged with conspiring to dump toxic waste at sea under a faked licence. [95]

■Waste dumped in a quarry near Bampton in Devon was found to have leaked out of the tip and there were fears that the River Exe might become contaminated. [96] A borehole examination revealed a massive leakage of oil through the rock strata and analysis of the water showed the concentration of heavy metals to be increasing. Devon's county geologist was uniquivocal about the unsuitability of the site for further use. 'It leaks', he said.[97] Haul Waste, the owners of the site, were subsequently refused a licence to continue tipping in the quarry – a decision which was overruled on appeal. In the mid-1970s, the site had been listed as one of the 53 tips in Britain most likely to pollute local water supplies.

■A tip – known locally as the 'bubbling cauldron' – at Ravensfield in South Yorkshire, was hurriedly fenced off after children were burned by acid fumes. Sludges which had leached were powerful enough to have corroded drums. The site had been in use for 20 years and a variety of wastes were indiscriminately dumped. Tars in the tip were found to contain up to 32 per cent of concentrated sulphuric acid, and investigations revealed that alkaline and acid wastes had been dumped within inches of each other. If they had combined the results could have been fatal. No one knew what wastes had been dumped (10,000 tons of contaminated materials were eventually treated) and for several months it proved impossible to trace the owner of the site. The then county waste disposal officer, John Holmes, told *Municipal Engineering*: 'Ravensfield is not the only private tip in this condition. There must be hundreds. I expect many more will be discovered.'[98]

■After an explosion at the Coalite chemical factory in Bolsover in 1968, waste contaminated with dioxin was dumped at a secret site in Derbyshire. Much of the waste is now thought to have been buried in a former open-cast mine near the village of Morton and just 100 yards from a local hospital. In 1976, Derbyshire County Council's then chief scientific officer, Joe Markland, concluded in a secret report that there was no need for public alarm over the site. Yet, as Catherine Caufield and Fred Pearce reported in *New Scientist*, 'Markland himself did not know where the dioxin was buried. He had, therefore, to rely on the assurances from the chairman of Coalite, Ted Needham, about, for example, the impermeability of the disposal site which, the report noted, "was said to have a clay bottom." '[99] Although Markland warned that it was unlikely that the dioxin would have been broken down by biological action, Neil Ashcroft, chief executive of the council, told Dennis Skinner MP in 1980 that 'it is very likely that the dioxin will have decomposed by now.' The same claim was made by the Severn-Trent Water Authority (STWA) which also deceived local villagers by telling them that any possible contamination of water supplies would be detected. Six months after that assurance, David Young of the STWA told Morton Paris Council: 'We do not carry out any analysis for dioxin.' It has also emerged that Ashcroft misled Skinner by telling him, in 1976, that the county council itself had decided to keep the location of the site secret. Ashcroft has since admitted to *New Scientist* that he lied on this point: the decision was in fact taken by council officers – not the elected representatives. When, in 1981, the council's Finance and General Purposes Committee ratified that previous decision, it did so without having seen the Markland report or apparently knowing where the dioxin was dumped.[100] In February 1982, a tribunal of inquiry set up by the council ruled that the dioxin dump could prove 'a severe hazard'.[101]

■For the villagers of Morton, however, the problem does not end there. Right next to the suspected dioxin dump is a toxic waste tip operated by Cambro Ltd. From the moment the tip opened in 1978 (after pressure was exerted by local industry on both Derbyshire County Council and the Yorkshire Water Authority) the tip was monitored by an environmental action group. 'It was discovered that the company was not accurately recording all the waste it accepted', reported Caufield and Peace. 'Among the "ghost" deliveries was a load of sodium nitrate (banned under the tip's licence) which Cambro recorded as a non-toxic iron compound, and trichloroethylene (also banned) was wrongly described as a solid aromatic hydrocarbon.'[102] In March 1981, Cambro was ordered to stop pumping water out of the tip into nearby streams after it was found to be contaminated with phenolic elements. Yet local residents 'saw the pump operating on weekends' – a time when the tip was supposed to be closed and when the tip operators could be confident of not receiving any official inspections.'[103] In February 1982, Derbyshire County Council ordered the tip to close – although local residents fear the decision will be reversed on appeal.[104]

How many of those incidents were accidental and how many the result of premeditated abuse, we shall never know. Reading through the literature, however, one cannot help but be struck at the paucity of our knowledge on the practice of landfill tipping and its attendant dangers. On the precautions that *should* be taken to prevent water pollution from a toxic dump, the Key Committee remarked: 'At the moment this is largely a matter of "hunch", which is hardly good enough in a scientific age.'[105] With that degree of ignorance, it is perhaps no surprise that the system is abused.

Yet the authorities – and not just the waste disposal industry – continue to deny the dangers. The Department of the Environment, for instance, claims that landfill is our safest means of waste disposal. It points to a 1978 study by the Institute of Geological Sciences which concluded that 'an ultra-cautious approach to landfill of hazardous and other types of waste is unjustified'.[106] But, it must be said, the £1.7 million study was only commissioned because, just two years earlier, the institute had warned that some 53 sites in Britain presented a 'theoretically serious risk to aquifers' and that they ought to be classed as 'high risk'.[107] So what lay behind the sudden change of opinion? Critics point out that the new study investigated no more than 19 'typical' sites – a tiny fraction of the total number in Great Britain – and that of those 19, only 15 were studied in depth. Even so, 2 sites were found to be causing water pollution. Moreover, the suggestion that the sites selected were 'representative' of the main geological types in the United Kingdom is perhaps misleading. Varying topography, rainfall patterns, soil differences and numerous other factors make each site unique and hence generalisation impossible.

'The report is far from reassuring', Brian Cope, a member of two government working parties on waste management, told me. 'The evidence from other countries is that pollution from landfill is almost inevitable, but in Britain no one has really looked for it.' He points to a survey conducted in the USA: out of 50 sites investigated, 43 showed migration of one or more hazardous substances: 40 showed migration of heavy metals; 30 of selenium, arsenic or cyanide: and 27 showed migration of organic chemicals. 'My understanding of the laws of science is that they apply as forcefully in Britain as they do in the

United States. I don't believe that toxic wastes behave differently just because they are American.'[108]

One site which has caused particular concern is the giant dump at Pitsea on the Essex Marshes. Lying on the Thames Estuary, just across the river from Canvey Island, Pitsea became one of Britain's largest hazardous waste dumps after the passing of the Deposit of Poisonous Waste Act. The Act which tightened restrictions on toxic waste disposal, resulted in an eightfold increase in the volume of chemicals being tipped at Pitsea in just three years.[109] Yet the site was not given a geological survey until 1973 – by which time it was one of Britain's largest disposal sites, taking waste from all over the country.

That survey proved somewhat embarrassing for the then owners, Redland-Purle (now called Cleanaway Ltd.) who had always assumed that Pitsea lay above an impermeable clay bowl into which chemicals could be safely poured. In fact, it was learned that the site formed a clay wedge, rather like a slice of cake laid on its side, which sloped down to the Thames Estuary. It thus appeared that the company's dumping operations threatened the whole estuary with massive pollution since the chemicals would simply dribble down the wedge into the river.[110]

In the event, Pitsea was exonerated after a study by the company's consultant geologist, Rod Aspinwall, showed that soils beneath the site had an unusual capacity to absorb and dilute chemicals.[111] Nonetheless, four years later, it was discovered that chemicals had leached into a nearby creek. In 1978, Aspinwall reported that leachate problems were continuing, and the local water authorities confirmed that leachate was flowing into an underground aquifer.[112] For its part, the local district council of Basildon wrote to Redland-Purle's solicitors expressing concern that 'the land is not suitable for the reception of inorganic wastes in unlimited quantities'.[113]

At odds with both Essex County Council and Redland-Purle over the safety of the site, Basildon District Council approached the House of Lords' Select Committee on Science and Technology who agreed to look into the problems. During the Committee's hearings, the Essex County Council and the Anglian Water Authority presented evidence that leachate from Pitsea was 'indistinguishable from that produced at a site receiving only domestic refuse' and that no trace of hazardous waste had been found.[114] That evidence was challenged by Brian

Cope. Pointing out that 'the composition of leachate changes with time and that analytical data on spot sampling have limited value,' he went on to comment: 'it would seem to me incredible to suggest that leachate from (hazardous) wastes has a similar chemical composition to domestic refuse leachate . . . you may wish to consider whether Essex County Council's interpretation of these results stems from ignorance of the scientific factors or from some other reason.'[115]

In the event, the Committee came down on the side of Essex County Council, arguing that Cope's evidence was 'sometimes tendentious and sometimes not scientifically substantiated'.[116] But although it acknowledged that the Pitsea had been badly managed in the past ('The Committee feel certain that, in the past at least, Basildon had good reason for suspicion about operations at Pitsea and they are very conscious of Essex County Council's statement that the site was "not good" in 1974 which was presumably an understatement') and warned that 'such impermeable linings (as clay) have not been in use long enough yet for anyone to be confident of their permanence' it none-theless stated that it could not agree with Basildon that Pitsea was being 'operated without due regard to public concern and safety'.[119] On the contrary, it felt the site was now being operated 'responsibly'.

But whereas the Select Committee gave Pitsea a clean bill of health, it had little good to say about the new regulations introduced by the DOE in 1981 in order to tighten up controls on dumping. Not least among the worries of the Select Committee is the way in which the DOE has chosen to define the 'toxicity' of a given waste. Indeed that definition – that 'a dose of not more than five cubic centimetres would be likely to cause death or serious damage to tissue if ingested by a child of 20 kilograms body weight or exposure to it for 15 minutes would be likely to cause serious damage to human tissue'[120] – has been described as 'a legal and scientific minefield' and virtually 'unenforceable' in a court of law.[121] It is also pointed out that the definition takes no heed of either the damage a waste might cause to the environment or of its sublethal and delayed effects.[122] Moreover, because the new regulations have cut by two thirds the number of wastes that are 'notifiable', there are fears that cowboy operators will return in force. It is, for example, possible to short-circuit the system by mixing 'notifiable' wastes with 'non-notifiable' wastes, thus escaping the need to inform the authorities about their disposal.[123]

Fears that the regulations will prove a cowboys charter are real enough. The Select Committee itself acknowledges that it is impossible to stamp out fly-tipping. Meanwhile, many in industry believe that the cowboys are already back. As Dr Arthur Coleman who runs three waste treatment plants under the name of Re-Chem told *New Scientist*: 'We lost one contract for incinerating cutting fluid recently. The company said the fluid was going to a plant in Cambridgeshire for recycling. I know what's in the fluid and I don't believe there is anything worth recycling. And as far as we can discover there isn't a recovery plant anywhere in Cambridgeshire anyway . . . in the last year (1981) we've lost 15 per cent of our business. Some of this is due to the recession, but a lot more is due to industry switching back to landfill and cutting corners.' [124]

What then of the future? If the evidence from the United States is anything to go by, the picture is far from reassuring. Faced with the increasing costs of legal disposal, many companies appear to be resorting to crime in order to get rid of their wastes. Illegal dumping is now on the increase and often is only discovered after the event – by which time contamination may be massive. In one incident, for example, a New Jersey policeman questioned a tanker driver who had almost finished emptying his load down a sewer. The officer became suspicious when his shoes began to disintegrate after he stepped into a puddle. [125]

Events such as this led the New Jersey State Legislature to set up a special department to investigate midnight hauliers and to place the waste disposal industry under surveillance. The department, which has brought numerous cases of illegal dumping to court was first headed by Edwin Stier, director of the State Division of Criminal Justice, a veteran investigator of organised crime and one of those responsible for exposing the extent of political corruption in the state. By and large, it appears that the companies involved take wastes perfectly legally – often fronting as recycling firms – and then dispose of them illicitly. In one case, a company was alleged to have connected metal pipes directly from its processing plant into the sewer system. The company, Scientific Chemicals, had been under surveillance for nearly six months and when police finally raided its premises, they caught a truck driver redhanded dumping some 5,000 gallons of untreated chemical wastes into a sewer. The company was charged with disposing of over 100,000 gallons of acid wastes, flammable solvents and untreated cyanide illegally. [126] In another incident, a waste disposer was charged with having dumped 55-gallon drums of untreated chemicals on derelict building sites in the city of Newark. The drums were thrown into pits dug by bulldozers and then covered roughly with earth. [127]

Many – particularly truckers – see the hand of organised crime behind the present wave of illegal dumping. They point out that whoever is in charge of the industry, the activities of midnight hauliers are now organised with the precision of military operations. In the past, it was usually left to waste disposal firms to make their own private deals with drivers they could trust to get rid of difficult cargoes with the minimum of questions asked. Today the arrangements are made by 'brokers' who employ their own truckers to carry out the job. Indeed, the rates paid are so good that some drivers make their living entirely by illegal dumping – and those wishing to join the club are strictly vetted. 'It is common talk among truckers that the brokers represent organised crime' says Andrew Schneider of Associated Press. [128]

Typically, a driver meets his 'broker' at a wayside café or in a lay-by. There he will be given the name of the company from which he is to pick up the waste; removable 'hazardous cargo' stickers and fake company insignia; a phoney manifest showing that he is carrying some harmless product; and the name of a contact who will show him where to discharge his lethal chemical cargo. From then on, the procedure is relatively simple: the driver picks up his load perfectly legitimately, filling in all the appropriate forms and signing a legal manifest for a cargo of chemical wastes. Once outside his client's factory, however, he removes all signs showing that he is carrying chemical wastes and substitutes the phoney manifest for the legal one. He then drives to his rendezvous, dumps the wastes and continues on to a second rendez-vous where he will pick up his pay. Even if he is stopped before he dumps his cargo, it is unlikely that police will search his truck.

As yet, the methods of British dumpers are not as sophisticated as their American counterparts. But will they become so? Few in the waste disposal industry would deny that fly-tipping continues apace and many fear that the practice will become more widespread as the present economic recession bites deeper. If that proves the case, then illegal dumpers will have a heyday – and organised crime will inevitably exploit the situation.

So long as ecological considerations play second fiddle to economic ones, the Department of the Environment will always be caught between the devil and the deep blue sea. Whichever way it turns, it cannot win – and it is the rest of us who will suffer. In the short term, we may avoid bankruptcies, but what about the future? How safe are we from the chemicals we have dumped over the last forty years? Where will the wastes we produce tomorrow be dumped? At what stages do we decide that our land is too valuable to be used as a coffin for chemicals we cannot handle? And when industry can only remain solvent by contaminating our environment, isn't the industrial game really up? For, ultimately, doesn't the solution lie in not generating wastes we do not know what to do with? As one incinerator operator put it to me: 'Cutting back on industrial activities might put me out of business, but it would eradicate the problem, wouldn't it?'

3
RADIATION:
HOW LOW CAN YOU GET?

THE ATOMIC bombs dropped on Nagasaki and Hiroshima in August 1945, provided a horrifying demonstration of the powers of ionising radiation – powers that few men could even have contemplated. It wasn't just the appalling physical destruction – buildings flattened for miles – that shocked American troops when they entered the two cities two weeks later, but rather the gruesome evidence that large doses of radiation could cause such untold biological damage. Today that damage has been well researched. We know that at 500 rems, most humans die; at 300 rems, the body's immunological system is grossly impaired; at 100 rems, nausea, vomiting and nosebleeds – the signs of radiation sickness – occur.[1] And more often than not, those who survive such high doses are condemned to suffer lingering deaths from leukemia and other cancers.

But whilst we know more than enough about the dangers of high doses of radiation, the authorities have consistently denied that low doses can cause significant biological harm. To be sure, the maximum permissible exposure limits for those working with radiation have been dramatically reduced since the early days of radiation research: from 73 rems in the late 1920s, to 50 rems in 1938, 25 rems in 1948, 15 in 1954 and, finally, to 5 rems in 1958.[2] That standard still remains in force, although the International Commission on Radiological Protection is now campaigning to raise the limits for exposure of certain organs.

The 5 rem limit is largely based on extrapolating from studies of cancer rates among those who survived the atomic bombs. Central to the argument is the notion that the effects of ionising radiation are directly proportional to the dose received. That assumption is now questioned by many eminent epidemiologists and radiation researchers. 'From 1960 to the present, an overwhelming amount of data has been accumulated that show there is no safe level of exposure and there is no dose of radiation so low that the risk of malignancy is zero,' writes Professor Karl Morgan, 'therefore, the question is not: is there a risk from low level exposure? Or what is the safe level of exposure? The question is how great is that risk?'[3] Indeed, Morgan has come to believe that in some cases small doses of radiation may actually be more harmful than large ones.[4]

Morgan's views find little favour in the nuclear industry. If he and his colleagues are correct, then exposure levels may have to be reduced so far that many existing nuclear plants would have to be closed down, or, at least, radically redesigned. Moreover, the industry would be faced with a flood of compensation claims from both former workers and those living near nuclear facilities, who have developed cancer after being exposed to radiation within supposedly 'acceptable' limits. Not surprisingly, then, those who challenge the official view that low-dose radiation is harmless have found themselves singled out for vicious attacks on their professional and personal integrity, while their research has been consistently ignored and suppressed.

But concern over 'low-dose' radiation is nothing new. It stems back to the very earliest days of nuclear experimentation. Between 1948 and 1962, the US Department of Defense carried out 183 above ground atomic bomb tests. Those tests were performed primarily in the Marshall Islands in the Pacific Ocean, and on the Nevada test site just north-west of Las Vegas. More than 200,000 soldiers were involved in the programme. Some were stationed as close as 2,500 yards from ground zero – the point at which a bomb is exploded – and expected to move into positions less than 200 yards from the site of the blast within minutes of the bomb being detonated.[5] The authorities maintain to this day that the soldiers involved in the tests only received low-level radiation. That being the case, they argue, none of them could have come to any harm as a direct result.

That claim is perhaps not surprising, for from the moment that the bomb tests were originally conceived the Department of Defense

(DOD) and the Atomic Energy Commission (AEC) – the body which 'umpired' the tests – took a deliberate decision not to disclose the dangers. The diary of the AEC's chairman at the time reveals that President Dwight Eisenhower personally ordered a propaganda campaign to 'keep the public confused about fission'.[6] It would appear that the campaign was successful, for the tests had a carnival atmosphere to them: indeed, busloads of spectators, including school-children, were taken on special outings to watch the bombs exploding.[7] As for the soldiers who took part in the tests, few remember being told about even the most basic precautions they should take to protect themselves against the blast. 'We saw the exercises as a holiday,' one soldier told me. 'They were a relief from the drudgery of the barracks. We had no idea what to expect. But when the bomb went off it was as if the bowels of hell had opened up. It was horrific.'[8]

'Just before they detonated the bomb, they told us to turn around and put our hands over our eyes,' recalls another soldier. 'When it went off, we felt an almost unbearable heat, like backing up to a fire with tight Levis on. We could see the bones in our hands through our closed eyelids, as if we were taking a big X-ray. Then they told us to turn around and watch the bomb. We saw the fireball go off, and the shock waves knocked several of us off our feet. The others hung on to each other to stay up. It was like being in winds of eighty miles per hour. The ground was shaking like it was an earthquake.'[9]

Today, thousands of the soldiers who were exposed to the bomb tests are suffering from blood and bone marrow diseases, cancers of those tissues most sensitive to radiation, respiratory disease and sterility. Nor are they the only ones to have been affected: 170,000 civilians living downwind from the bomb test site in Nevada were exposed to fallout, and radioactive dust thrown up into the upper atmosphere by the blast was deposited back on earth as far away as New York. Recent studies show a threefold increase in the cancer rate of children exposed to fallout from the tests.[10]

Those in the Marshall Islands fared even worse. After the first atomic tests, the Marshallese were evacuated by the US authorities because their islands were considered 'radioactive deserts'. Those evacuations did not last long, however, and by 1957, the inhabitants of some of the major atolls in the Marshalls had been allowed to return to their homelands. Internal documents reveal that the agency knew that at least one atoll, Rongelap, was still contaminated with radiation at levels ten times higher than in other parts of the world. Even so, it let the native Marshallese return. At the time, an AEC scientist wrote in a memorandum: 'The habitation of these people on the island will afford most valuable ecological radiation data on human beings.'[11] By 1964, 19 out of the 21 Rongelap children who were aged under twenty-one in 1954 had developed thyroid cancer.[12]

That element of wilful experimentation had been present throughout the whole test programme. Indeed, the Department of Defense made it clear that one aim of the bomb tests was to see how soldiers would react when exposed to the full horrors of an atomic blast. 'Can a highly trained soldier think clearly and perform the duties of his fighting mission efficiently in a shadow of a nuclear bomb's mushroom cloud?' asks a DOD press release at the time of the 'Smoky' test programme. 'Two minutes after a blast with an explosive force of over 20,000 tons of TNT will his hands tremble as he kneels to field-strip and reassemble his rifle? Will he obey the orders of his commanding officer, or will he falter as the choking dust cloud whirls around him? Will he move quickly to clear a minefield or will he "gawk" at the eerie snowcap forming above his head? For the first time since man learned to split the atom, the United States army is prepared to find the answers to these and other unknowns concerning human behaviour in nuclear warfare.'[13]

The army was simply using its soldiers as human guinea pigs with no regard at all for their safety or any possible side effects. When it became clear that those side effects were severe, public outrage forced the US Department of Defense into an extremely difficult position. It extricated itself by freezing all the relevant records and adamantly denying any responsibility. Soldiers who later developed cancer found themselves stonewalled when they tried to obtain the radiation records which would have enabled them to claim compensation. And even government authorities looking into the problem were obstructed in their research. In late November 1975, for instance, a doctor working at the Veterans Administration Hospital in Salt Lake City, Utah, learned of a patient who had developed acute myelocytic leukemia.[14] The patient had taken part in Operation Smoky and the doctor decided to contact the Centre for Disease Control to see if they could unearth a possible link. The CDC, a branch of the Department of

Health, Education and Welfare, was extremely interested and agreed to undertake a study of former Smoky veterans to determine their incidence of leukemia and other cancers. The first problem for the CDC team, headed by Dr William Foege and Dr Glyn Caldwell, was to find out how much radiation the soldiers had been exposed to. But when they contacted the Department of Defense's Armed Forces Radiobiology Research Unit they were told that such information could only be given if they could supply the names of the soldiers involved in the tests. Those names were by no means easy to track down. And the task was made more difficult by the Department of Defense's apparent inability to supply even a list of army units present at the Smoky explosion.

That list was eventually obtained when Caldwell telephoned the General Electric Corporation and was put in touch with an independent computer bank which did contract work for the Department of Defense. They immediately supplied the names of all the units involved. Not that the Department of Defense did not have access to the information; indeed, they supplied a duplicate to Caldwell a few months later.[15] Despite this foot-dragging on the part of the authorities, the CDC completed its study in 1978. The leukemia rate amongst Smoky veterans was found to be two times higher than that in a normal population.[16]

Intrigued by those results and alarmed by a seeming excess of leukemias in several counties downwind of the Nevada test site, Dr Joseph Lyon, a doctor at the University of Utah's College of Medicine, conducted a limited epidemiological survey. He found a threefold increase in leukemia deaths amongst children exposed to fallout.[17]

Joseph Lyon's survey was not the first to have found such an effect. Documents released under the Freedom of Information Act reveal that, in 1965, a similar study had been undertaken by Dr Edward Weiss of the US Public Health Service's Division of Radiological Health. That study had found a doubling of the leukemia rate but had been suppressed by the Atomic Energy Commission.[18]

Also suppressed was a report on a sudden outbreak of spontaneous abortions, deaths and birth defects among sheep grazing the grasslands beneath the path of the fallout from the bomb tests. The sheep had been contaminated by radiation from a series of 'dirty' bombs exploded in the early fifties. The description 'dirty' is applied because the bombs were detonated almost at ground level – from platforms 300 feet high – and consequently the radioactive dust clouds they created were carried for miles in the tornado-force winds the explosion triggered off. No sooner had researchers from the Public Health Service (PHS) started their investigation of the so-called 'sheep incident', than they were visited by a senior AEC representative who suggested, none too subtly, that radiation could not possibly be the cause of the strange plague hitting sheep flocks. The official went on to threaten that, unless the AEC was presented with a report that came to similar conclusions, funds might dry up for further research.[19] The very same day, the PHS scientists sent in their report. There was no connection, it stated, between the sheep deaths and birth defects – which had affected a quarter of the flocks in the area – and the atomic bomb tests being conducted in Nevada. In 1982, several sheep farmers sued the US government for damages.[20]

By 1979, the controversy over the fate of the veterans exposed to the atomic bomb tests in the fifties had reached such a pitch that the US government appointed a special 'task force' to examine their case. The task force maintained the fiction that the soldiers had been exposed to low doses of radiation, quoting Department of Defense radiation statistics to prove their point. 'The DOD's reconstruction of events at the atmospheric tests suggests that radiation exposures were quite low, because of the radiation safety procedures used at the tests,' argues the report. 'It is currently estimated that about 90 per cent of the [soldiers participating] in the tests received less than 1 rem; and about 97 per cent received less than 3 rems.'[21] Those levels are, of course, well within the 5 rem standard currently accepted as safe by the International Commission on Radiological Protection, but what the task force omitted to say was that few of the soldiers even had radiation badges to monitor their exposure.[22] And those that did had them collected by their officers for 'processing' before they were registered on any official files. 'The report was written to give the Veterans Administration grounds for denying compensation to veterans of the nuclear weapons tests,' claims Dr Irwin Bross, an outspoken critic of current radiation standards. 'To this end, the report suppresses new evidence of radiation hazards and disparages the scientists who have done these studies.'[23, 24]

With the estimated cost of compensation claims from veterans approaching the $5 billion mark, the motive for the US government's consistent attempts to deny responsibility are clear. That they should have been supported in their attempts by the Atomic Energy Commission – and later the Department of Energy – was also predictable. For by now, a crop of incidents involving workers in the nuclear industry had thrown the whole 5 rem standard into doubt – and whilst the army only had its short-term future at stake if the standard was lowered, the nuclear industry felt that its life was in jeopardy.

Joe Harding worked for eighteen years at a uranium enrichment plant, owned by the Union Carbide Corporation of Peduccah, Kentucky. He was to have testified at a series of hearings held in April 1980 by the pressure group, Citizens Hearings on Radiation Victims, but he died a month before. His widow and daughter took the witness stand in his place. 'They never told my husband that radiation was harmful,' said Mrs Harding, her voice trembling. 'They told him that it would hurt him no more than a luminous dial wristwatch. And now he's dead.'[25]

A day before he died, Harding completed a taped interview with Pierre Fruhling, a Swedish journalist.[26] The tapes describe in harrowing detail the working conditions at the enrichment plant. 'There was uranium dust all over the floor, so deep that you could see the footprints in it. We wore film badges to monitor our radiation dose; they were collected once a month and sent to Oak Ridge Laboratory, also run by Union Carbide's Nuclear Division, for analysis, but we never heard the results. One time, three or four of us laid our film badges on top of a smoking chuck of uranium for eight hours. Still we didn't hear from them.'

Although the cylinders of enriched uranium being shipped from the plant were regularly monitored for excessive radiation levels, Harding alleges that those tests were constantly falsified. 'On one occasion, a cylinder I surveyed showed levels too 'hot' for shipment. I reported to the supervisor but he told me: "Listen, we already got this cylinder checked in on this truck. So let's get a real good reading and get it shipped." '

By the time he died, twenty-seven years after he was first employed at the plant, Joe Harding was a virtual skeleton. In 1965, most of his stomach was removed. In 1979, a massive tumour was scraped from his thigh. And, perhaps most disturbing of all, nail-like growths had begun sprouting from the backs of his hands, his wrists, elbows and shoulders. Various doctors believe that these growths were the result of spontaneous cell mutations.

Surprisingly, local Peduccah doctors never made a positive diagnosis of Harding's early stomach cancers. The symptoms were described in detail in all his medical reports, but no explanation was given for them. 'When Joe first went to his local doctor, he was told he had radiation damage,' his widow recalls. 'But the doctor wouldn't put it in writing. He just wrote that the cause of Joe's stomach problems was unknown.' In fact, Mrs Harding alleges that Union Carbide threatened to sue one doctor who was bold enough to suggest that Joe Harding's illness was radiation-induced. 'That's how powerful Union Carbide is in Peduccah. They just put the doctors off. Finally we had to go to an out-of-town doctor to get treatment.'

That Union Carbide should be so keen to deny the connection between Joe Harding's death and his work with uranium is perhaps not surprising. Despite working most of his life under the 5 rem regime, Joe had suffered almost the entire range of radiation-induced cancer. To admit responsibility for his death would inevitably bring the 5 rem standard into question, opening the floodgates for a spate of compensation claims from other nuclear workers who had died of cancer. Moreover, with the near meltdown at Three Mile Island still very much in mind, the nuclear industry must have been aware that any apparent admission that radiation could cause death at doses lower than those publicly admitted to be safe raised the possibility that those living near nuclear facilities might also sue for possible damage to their health.

Already, studies by Dr Ernest Sternglass had shown an alarming correlation between cancer rates in areas neighbouring nuclear reactors and the radiation released from those reactors. Sternglass found, for instance, that the rates of leukemia in those living near the Shippingport reactor in Pennsylvania rose by 70 per cent in the first ten years of the reactor's operation. The leukemia rate in Pennsylvania as a whole rose by only 7 per cent during the same period. That correlation has been confirmed by other studies, the most recent being that conducted by the Bremen Institute for Biological Safety. 'The institute found that in the ten years before the Lingen reactor near Nieder-sachsen, West Germany, began operation, the surrounding population experienced only 30 leukemia deaths,' report Jim Garrison and Claire Ryle of the Radiation and Health Information Service. 'In the ten years after the reactor began operations, however, the same population suffered 230 leukemia deaths, 170 of which were to children under the age of fifteen.'[27]

When the Shippingport study first appeared in 1973, Sternglass found himself the focus of harassment by the nuclear industry. Much the same treatment has been meted out to other critics of present exposure standards:

■'Back in 1969,' recalls Dr Arthur Tamplin, now of the National Resources Defense Council, 'my colleague, John Gofman, and I became critical of radiation exposure standards. We had been listened to with deference within the Atomic Energy Commission for so long that we decided to go public and we presented our findings to a scientific meeting in San Francisco. After that, all hell broke out. I had a group at that time at (the Lawrence Livermore) laboratory of thirteen people. Within a short period of time the group was cut down to two people and then the other person was fired. Also, there was an effort on the part of the laboratory to censor a report that I was going to present to the American Association for the Advancement of Science meeting. Because the press had got so interested in the whole controversy, the laboratory was clearly embarrassed about . . . firing Gofman and me. Gofman had a research programme on chromosomes and cancer which was about a $250,000 a year programme. That was cut off. Gofman left the laboratory. But I stayed on . . . essentially as a non-person. I had no assignments but I had an office and I could get my pay check every month but I was never given any assignment in the laboratory. I stayed on because I thought it was a necessary irritant and embarrassment to the Atomic Energy Commission.'[28]

■'I didn't run into any serious problems until shortly before the time I was to retire from Oak Ridge National Laboratory,' says Professor Karl Morgan. 'In July 1971, I had sent ahead to Nuremburg, Germany, 200 copies of a paper I was to deliver there. I was on vacation in Switzerland for a week. When I went to the airport in Zurich, the girl at the desk said excitedly, "there have been numerous phone calls for you. Get to a phone as quickly as you can." She gave me the number, a number in the States. Dr Peller, the assistant director of Oak Ridge National Laboratory came to the phone. He said . . . they had looked at my paper again and found that some changes had to be made in it. He instructed persons in the laboratory to delete certain parts and he had wired the authorities in Nuremburg to throw the 200 advance copies away and to replace them by this (edited version) which had certain sections and pages torn out of it. The paper showed that some types of reactor were safer than others. It showed that the thermal breeder system we were interested in at the laboratory was, according to my calculations, some 270 times safer than the liquid metal fast breeder system which shortly afterward became the only egg in our basket. [29]

■Dr Irwin Bross of Rosewell Park Memorial Hospital, New York, had his funds cut off after publishing the results of a survey which showed that children who had been X-rayed in the womb had a three to four times higher risk of developing leukemia than those who had not been X-rayed. [30]

■Dr Thomas Najarian, a doctor at the Veterans Administration Hospital in Boston, found that nearly 38.5 per cent of workers at the Portsmouth Naval Shipyard in New Hampshire died of cancer. That figure compares with an average rate of 21.7 per cent for workers at shipyards not handling nuclear materials and 18 per cent for the general American population. The rate of leukemias was 450 per cent higher than average and their largest incidence was found amongst workers whose average yearly radiation dose was 4 rems – one rem below the permitted maximum whole body dose. Moreover, older workers appear worst affected – 60 per cent of those aged between sixty and sixty-nine dying of various cancers. [31]

Najarian, who stressed to me that he is not opposed to nuclear power, became interested in the problem when a young patient he was treating for leukemia mentioned that many of his workmates were suffering from the disease or had died young. When Najarian approached the US army for the radiation exposure records of workers in the shipyard, he was refused access to the information. Undeterred, he turned to the *Boston Globe* for help. The newspaper took up his cause and provided him with five reporters to lend a hand in sifting through some 100,000 death certificates. From those, Najarian identified 1,722 former shipyard workers together with their cause of death. The *Globe* also filed a suit against the navy under the Freedom of Information Act in order to force the authorities to release the radiation data.

Prompted by that court case, Senator Thomas McIntyre called on the Centre for Disease Control to conduct a thorough survey of the workers' health – and initially it would appear that the navy agreed to the plan. By the end of February 1978, a month after Najarian had published his initial findings in the *Globe,* McIntyre learned that the navy had refused the CDC access to its radiation exposure files and was insisting that the study be undertaken by the Department of Defense. 'There are growing suspicions that the Pentagon is trying to stonewall efforts by the CDC to determine if there is a problem at the shipyards,' McIntyre told a Senate committee. 'In this climate of suspicion and distress the navy has a clear obligation to cooperate, to stop obstructing the CDC and to start being candid with shipyard workers.'[32]

Eventually, the navy agreed to cooperate in the CDC study but, even so, doubts have been expressed about the objectivity of the team of scientists chosen to oversee the project. By 1979, for instance, Dr Irwin Bross – a member of the team – accused the authorities of stalling the investigation 'at every turn' and of stacking the CDC team with pro-government scientists, many of whom were known for their view that low-dose radiation cannot cause biological harm. 'We are clearly in the middle of a serious cover-up,' Bross announced to the press. 'They just don't want the information out.'[33]

But perhaps the best documented – and certainly the most concerted – effort to cover up the hazards of low-dose radiation concerns a study undertaken at the Hanford nuclear facility in Washington State. Hanford is one of the main reprocessing plants in the United States, and, in 1964, Dr Thomas Mancuso of the University of Pittsburgh was asked by the Atomic Energy Commission to conduct a survey of cancer-rates amongst Hanford workers. Mancuso, whose research on the health hazards of chemical pollution had earlier established his reputation as one of America's foremost epidemiologists, undertook the study in good faith, firmly believing that the AEC was genuinely interested in furthering our knowledge of the dangers of radiation and in safeguarding the health of nuclear workers.

Documents released under the Freedom of Information Act, however, reveal a very different story.[34] Right from the start, the AEC's principal concern was that the study should both allay fears about the dangers of radiation and provide a useful weapon for fending off compensation claims by former workers who were dying of cancer. 'It seems highly probable that if one went through the mechanics of calculating the kinds of radiation effects which a study of the present magnitude might detect, one would be led to conclude that the undertaking is a hopeless one,' wrote Professor William Schull, a consultant to the AEC. 'However, as earlier recognised, it may have other merit in that it may provide a firmer basis for settlement of claims against the AEC . . . and a buttress against ill-conceived and opportunistic claims which might be levelled against the AEC.'[35]

Schull's attitude was echoed by virtually every other AEC consultant involved in the study. Thus, Professor Brian MacMahon of Harvard University: 'In my opinion this study does not have, never did have, and never (in any practical sense) will have, any possibility of contributing to knowledge of radiation effects in man . . . I recognise that much of the motivation for starting this study arose from the "political" need for assurance that AEC employees are not suffering harmful effects.'[36]

Or, again, in a memorandum to S.G. English, the AEC's assistant general manager for research, from John Totter, director of the AEC's division of biology and medicine: 'The study probably will not confirm or refute any important hypotheses but should permit a statement to the effect that a careful study of workers in the industry has disclosed no harmful effects of radiation (if the results are negative as they are likely to be). The statement, supported by appropriate documentation, would seem to justify the existence of the study. A corollary statement could presumably be made about other similarly exposed populations.'[37]

But if the AEC expected Mancuso to play ball and sacrifice his scientific integrity for politics, it was soon disappointed. The inevitable battle of wills came in 1974, when Dr Samuel Milham, an epidemiologist from the Washington Department of Health, reported that the cancer rate among workers at the Hanford plant was five times higher than expected. The AEC – which by now had been renamed the Department of Energy – immediately contacted Milham and asked him to hold off publishing his results. Milham agreed since he knew that the Mancuso study was nearing completion and because he respected Mancuso. A meeting was also set up between Mancuso's statistician, Dr Barkov Sanders, and Milham to discuss Milham's results. At the same time, the DOE sent Milham's data to the government-funded Batelle Pacific Northwest Laboratory for re-analysis.[38]

Far from finding Milham at fault, however, Batelle confirmed his results – to the obvious chagrin of the DOE. 'We hoped to get a good answer to the Milham report and, instead, it looks like we have support for it,' confided one official. The meeting between Sanders and Milham also failed to demolish Milham's findings. 'Much of the discussion at this meeting involved the details of the statistical method and other technical factors which were difficult to follow,' reports Mr Fasulo, a DOE officer who was present at the meeting. 'However, when I was able to bring the conversation around to more basic agreements and disagreements between Sanders and Milham, I was completely surprised to hear what sounded very much like apparent agreement between Sanders and Milham.'[39]

Realising that they were running out of cards to play against Milham, DOE officials then turned to Mancuso in the hope that he would publicly refute Milham's research. In June 1974, Dr Sidney Marks of the Energy Research and Development Agency contacted Mancuso and asked him to put his name to a press release repudiating Milham's findings. The press release claimed that Mancuso's data on Hanford indicated 'that 1) there was no apparent significant difference in radiation-related effects between Hanford employees and their siblings; and 2) based on scrutiny of some 4,000 death certificates, there was no evidence of cancer or other deaths attributable to ionising radiation occurring more often among Hanford workers than among other non-Hanford brothers and/or sisters.'[40] Knowing that his results were still inconclusive, Mancuso refused to put his name to such a categorical statement.[41] Almost immediately, his grant was terminated and ERDA bluntly informed him that the data he had accumulated was to be moved to a government research centre at Oak Ridge, Tennessee.[42]

The reason given by ERDA for the transfer was 'Mancuso's imminent retirement'.[43] In fact, Mancuso was only sixty-two years old at the time and under the University of Pittsburgh's retirement rules, he still had another eight years tenancy as a professor at the University's School of Public Health. When this was pointed out to ERDA, the then assistant administrator, Dr James Liverman, abruptly changed his tactics and argued that the real reason for Mancuso being taken off the project was that a peer review of his research had been highly critical of the procedures he was using. Dr Sidney Marks agreed – this despite having praised Mancuso for his 'meticulous data collection' and his 'extraordinary quality control'. Only one of the reviewers had explicitly recommended that Mancuso be replaced. Internal documents obtained under the Freedom of Information Act reveal that Marks' motives for criticising Mancuso and urging his dismissal were highly political. At the back of his mind was the fear that if Mancuso was removed after he had published positive findings, then there would be a public outcry. 'Overtures to [other] possible candidates must be carried out now in a clandestine atmosphere,' he urged his superiors in a memorandum.[45] Marks himself was later appointed to supervise the research programme.[46]

One reason Mancuso had been unwilling to put his name to the press release criticising Milham was that he was at the time extremely unsure of his own position. In fact, he was having difficulty making sense of Dr Sanders' statistical analysis, which seemed to imply that radiation was actually beneficial.[47] As a result he approached Dr Alice Stewart of Queen Elizabeth Hospital, Birmingham, to ask her if she would be kind enough to re-examine the data. Dr Stewart was on the Medical Advisory Committee to the Hanford project and was internationally renowned for her classic study in the fifties linking the X-raying of children in their mothers' wombs to an increase in the rate of childhood leukemias. Steward readily agreed to Mancuso's request on the condition that she could also employ Dr George Kneele of Oxford University as her statistician.[48]

In July 1976, Stewart and Kneele flew to America and began the reanalysis of Mancuso's data. It didn't take Stewart and Kneele long to unravel the mystery. Mancuso's study had been based on a comparison between exposed and non-exposed workers. But what it had failed to take into account was that the workers who were most exposed were young men specially selected for their physical fitness. Because that group was most resistant to the effects of radiation, and so had a lower casualty rate than older colleagues who were exposed to less radiation, the figures suggested that radiation actually increased the lifespan. Once the ages were taken into account, a very different picture emerged.[49]

Mancuso, Stewart and Kneele published their findings in late 1976. Their conclusions were startling: workers in the Hanford plant had an estimated 26 per cent higher risk of dying from cancer than that expected – and the risks of dying from some cancers, such as those of the bone marrow, were increased by 107 per cent. Those figures suggest that current radiation standards may be as much as ten times too high.[50]

Stewart was amazed by the often vitriolic personal attacks that followed the publication of the Hanford Data. In Britain, where she testified about her research at the public inquiry into the building of a Thermal Oxide Reprocessing Plant at Windscale, Mr Justice Parker devoted a considerable part of his report on her findings attacking her evidence as much on a personal as a rational basis. Even when he did deal with her scientific data, Parker ignored a set of new tables submitted by Stewart to clear up some of the points which he found unclear.[51] That treatment was particularly galling to Stewart who, when the inquiry was announced, had offered to give evidence on behalf of British Nuclear Fuels, the company that runs Windscale, in the belief that the nuclear industry would be genuinely concerned about the implications of the Hanford data and would bring the new reprocessing plant to stricter standards.[52] The subsequent behaviour of the authorities makes such a charitable view untenable.

Undoubtedly, the key to the nuclear industry's cover-up of the dangers of low-level radiation lies in the recognition that if the findings of researchers such as Mancuso, Stewart and Kneele are correct, then – as Justice Parker himself admitted – the whole future of civil nuclear power would be seriously jeopardised.[53] Quite simply, the cost of implementing their recommendations would be prohibitive. For that reason, the nuclear industry has deliberately distorted and suppressed vital evidence on the hazards of low-dose radiation. But the results of this deception, the rising cancer rates, and the inevitable genetic injury, will very soon be harder to conceal.

4
THE TRUTH ABOUT MICROWAVES

SCIENTISTS THE world over have only recently become aware of an invisible threat which is barely understood but growing daily. They call it 'electrical smog'.

Electrical smog is created by the thousands of electrical gadgets – from radar to satellites, television transmitters, microwave relay towers, microwave ovens, CB radios and high-voltage electricity lines – on which our modern way of life increasingly depends. Those devices inevitably create waves of electric and magnetic radiation whose strength and intensity is gauged along what physicists call the 'electromagnetic spectrum'. At the bottom end of the spectrum are extremely low-frequency (ELF) waves generated by, for example, high voltage power lines: at the opposite end are gamma rays. In between, in ascending order of frequency (a measure of how many times the waves vibrate each second) are microwaves, infra-red radiation, visible light, ultra-violet radiation and X-rays. Unlike gamma rays and X-rays, sources of low-frequency radiation are non-ionising – that is, they lack the ability to break up the material through which they pass into charged particles – and consequently they have long been considered benign, their only possible danger being their capacity to cause electric shocks and heat body tissue.

It was on the basis of this heating effect that the US authorities set a safety standard for exposure to low-frequency radiation of 10 milliwatts per square centimetre of exposed flesh, a figure that is one-tenth of the intensity at which microwaves are known to cause heat. Below that level – adopted as a standard throughout the West – low-frequency radiation is claimed to be harmless. Indeed, despite evidence to the contrary from animal experiments in the 1930s, scientists were so convinced that heating was the only danger from low-frequency radiation that one researcher, who found significant changes in the white blood cell counts of workers exposed to minute doses of micro-waves, dismissed the results as a laboratory error. [1]

Today, experts are less sanguine. Indeed, one US government report recently expressed fears that as our use of electronic technology mush-rooms, so electronic smog will become 'a more insidious threat to human health than even chemical pollution'. [2] That, perhaps, is an exaggeration; nonetheless, we would do well to remember that the average American now receives a daily dose of electromagnetic radiation 200 million times more intense than that taken in from natural sources such as the sun. [3] Meanwhile, there is a mounting tide of evidence that low-frequency radiation – at levels well below the 10 milliwatt standard – can cause health effects from decreased fertility to cataracts, cancer, genetic damage and birth defects. Those dangers, claims Paul Brodeur, author of the prize-winning book, *The Zapping of America*, have been deliberately hidden from the public. Why? What is it that the authorities know that the rest of us do not? And what exactly is the price we will have to pay for our ignorance?

In the early sixties, Dr Milton Zaret, an ophthalmologist now practising in Scarsdale, New York, was approached by agents from the Central Intelligence Agency. At first the questions seemed innocuous enough. Zaret, after all, was one of America's top specialists on the effects of microwaves on the human eye and there seemed nothing amiss in the CIA picking his brains on his latest research. It soon became clear, however, that the agency's interests were more than academic. Was it safe to use a new camera that took pictures at night with an invisible laser beam instead of a conventional flashbulb? Or would the laser beam damage the eye? Could a micro-wave beamed at the brain from a distance affect the way a person might act? Would a laser beam directed at a listening device be liable to injure anybody inside the room being bugged? And could micro-waves be used to break down prisoners under interrogation? [4]

Zaret was puzzled by the approach. Then, at another meeting with the CIA early in 1965, the cat finally slithered out of the bag. [5] The US embassy in Moscow was being irradiated with microwaves. Defence scientists were baffled: the Moscow Signal, as the microwave beam was code-named, appeared totally unsuitable for eavesdropping or for jamming the embassy's electronic surveillance equipment. So what was its purpose? Most intriguing of all, the beam was being transmitted at a mere 4 milliwatts per square centimetre – well within the US 10 milliwatt standard – but a level which the Russians had always claimed could cause biological damage and behavioural effects.[6] Was the Kremlin bluffing? Or had the Pentagon underestimated the power of microwaves? In which case, was the entire US defence system based on an exposure standard which could jeopardise national security?

Zaret suggested that the only way of finding out was to replicate the experiments carried out by Russian scientists and see if low levels of microwaves could indeed cause biological damage. That research was conducted by Zaret for the Advanced Research Projects Agency and by and large he was able to confirm the Soviet results. 'On one occasion,' he told Paul Brodeur, 'we not only succeeded in replicating a Czechoslovak study of behavioural effects in rats, but also observed some unique convulsions in the animals before they died.'[7] Soon after he reported this to his superiors at the Department of Defense, however, his research funds were cut off.[8] Later, he learned unofficially that similar results – never to be published – had been observed in experiments conducted as part of a top-secret programme at the Walter Reed Army Institute in Washington.[9] In fact, when the full story behind the Moscow Signal was finally made public, Zaret's worst fears were confirmed: not only were embassy officials suffering from an abnormally high rate of cancer and blood disorders, but – more disturbing still – a significant number of babies born to women working in the embassy were deformed, and serious genetic damage was observed in blood samples taken from four embassy employees.[10] Those dramatic revelations would not come for another ten years, however, for by 1965 the microwave cover-up was well and truly underway.

Zaret had already experienced attempts to suppress research which might have compromised the 10 milliwatt standard. In 1959, he had been part of a team investigating the incidence of cataracts and lens defects in the eyes of radar operators employed by the Department of Defense. Initially, the survey – known as the Tri-Service Programme – proved inconclusive. Some 1,600 workers employed at military and civilian bases throughout the US were examined but no cataracts were found and what lens damage was observed could be explained by the normal process of ageing. About this time, however, several large electronic companies – many of which were involved in Tri-Service – began to send Zaret employees who had developed cataracts for private treatment. 'I saw half a dozen cases in 1961 and 1962,' Zaret recalls. 'The patients were sent to me because there was a question as to whether they had been injured by microwave radiation. Of course, every one of them was a potential legal case, and it is to the credit of the companies that they continued to send those cases, for I made it clear that I would disclose my findings to each patient and I requested that I be permitted to perform follow-up examinations of them in the future. As things turned out, what I found ultimately changed my whole thinking about how microwaves cause cataracts.'[11]

Not only had all six patients developed full cataracts but, most significantly, the cataracts had formed on the back of the lens capsule – an extremely rare phenomenon and a symptom which Zaret soon came to recognise as 'the special signature' of overexposure to microwave radiation. 'Naturally, I began looking for similar abnormalities in the people who had been selected for the official survey and I soon found them,' he told Paul Brodeur. 'In one group of forty-odd radar trouble-shooters from a large electronics company, I found that fully one-third of them had roughening and thickening of the posterior capsular surface . . . By this time I was beginning to wonder about the military's attitude towards the problem of microwave exposure. Here, I had spent three years examining nearly 1,600 microwave workers and, except for one case that didn't count because diabetes was involved,* I hadn't come across a single cataract. Then, right in the middle of my survey, some of the very firms that were taking part in it began sending me patients on the side – patients who had been diagnosed as having cataracts. Why weren't such patients included in the official survey? Why did they all come from private companies? Why had I not seen any cataracts among military personnel? Had I been examining a true cross-section of people exposed to microwave radiation? Or was there something funny going on in the selection process, because of worries over public disclosure and possible legal problems?'[12]

---

* Diabetes is known to be a factor in the development of cataracts.

Zaret's findings were a direct threat to the 10 milliwatt standard which, by 1965, had been adopted by all branches of the armed services in the United States. As if to underline the point, the air force terminated their research contract and attempted to block any further investigation into the cataract problem.[13] By 1968, however, Zaret – working independently – had documented 42 cases of confirmed microwave cataracts and over 200 cases of scarring of the back of the lens capsule – a telltale sign of incipient damage.[14] Not that the military were impressed by his findings. 'There's no such thing as a microwave cataract,' he was brusquely told by Colonel Budd Appleton, chief ophthalmologist at the Walter Reed General Army Hospital.[15] Appleton claimed that the cataracts were simply the result of ageing – although he failed to explain why, in almost all of the 42 cases, the cataracts had only formed in one eye, whereas senile cataracts usually develop in both eyes.[16]

'Of course, the military people were anxious about my findings for a number of reasons,' Zaret told Paul Brodeur. 'First of all, if I turned out to be correct, and it became widely accepted that microwaves could cause specific and recognisable types of cataract, the armed forces were liable to incur some huge medico-legal problems, especially with civilian employees who had been exposed to radar. Second, and even more important, an enormous part of the nation's weapons development programme for the next ten years, including the antiballistic missile system, was predicted on the assumption that the 10 milliwatt level was safe. If this standard turned out to be unsafe and had to be lowered, the cost of relocating radar and missile sites, let alone redesigning equipment, would amount to billions of dollars. With so much at stake, the military could scarcely afford to accept any findings that cast any doubt on the theory that cataract formation was thermal in origin.'[17]

Today, Zaret goes further and alleges that he is blacklisted from receiving funds for research by the Department of Defense, the Food and Drugs Administration and the Environmental Protection Agency. Indeed, Zaret recently described government-sponsored research as nothing more than 'intelligent looks in the wrong direction'.[18] 'It's almost as if it has become anti-American to be against the 10 milliwatt standard,' he told a reporter from *Common Weal*, an environmental magazine. 'Most of the people involved in the research are now hacks – none of our good scientists are in the field. They find it too compromising.'[19]

The 10 milliwatt standard was based on the research of Dr Herman Schwan, a German scientist who came to America after the Second World War. He had based the figure on theoretical calculations using a metal ball as a model of a human being and then offsetting the heat absorbed by the ball against the heat lost by the normal processes of sweating.[20] Even Schwan, however, has described that rather rough and ready experiment as a crude measure of the power of microwaves and warned that the 10 milliwatt standard could prove 'insufficient protection' against the dangers of low-frequency radiation.[21] That criticism has been echoed by Dr Charles Susskind, professor of Electrical Engineering at the University of California at Berkeley, who told a 1968 Senate committee that few American scientists had even bothered to investigate the subtle biological effects of microwaves. He went on to brand the thermal theory (the supposition that heating was the only danger posed by low-frequency radiation) as a mere 'catechism'.[22]

In particular, Susskind berated the authorities for ignoring Soviet research which revealed biological effects at far lower levels of exposure than those tolerated in the United States. Indeed, since the 1930s, Soviet scientists recognised that microwaves could affect the central nervous system. Whereas the US military dismissed complaints by radar workers of headaches, eye pains and fatigue as 'subjective symptoms', the Russians were alarmed enough to conduct a full-scale epidemiological survey. That survey found that prolonged exposure to microwaves caused 'stabbing pains in the heart, dizziness, irritability, emotional instability, depression, diminished intellectual capacity, partial loss of memory, loss of appetite and loss of hair'.[23] It was also noted that microwaves could cause hallucinations and changes in white blood cell counts – a sign of leukemia. Indeed, the Russians took the dangers of low-frequency radiation so seriously that they set the safe exposure level for unprotected workers at 0.01 milliwatts per square centimetre – 1,000 times stricter than that in the United States. The standards laid down for civilians were 10,000 times more strict.[24]

Those Soviet standards should have alerted Western authorities to the possibility of more insidious effects from microwaves than mere heating. Not so. All government research was directed explicitly towards supporting the 10 milliwatt standard: witness a 1975 Pentagon report which urged that studies be undertaken 'to *disprove* electromagnetic radiation bioeffects'.[25] It need hardly be said that as the principal source of funds for microwave research, the Pentagon was able to achieve that aim by the simple expedient of terminating financial support for those research projects which jeopardised the 10 milliwatt standard. Nonetheless, Zaret and other scientists have been able to compile an impressive dossier of microwave-related injuries at levels well below 10 milliwatts:

■Arthur Kay was exposed to large doses of microwaves whilst working as a radar operator during the Korean War. Soon after his discharge, he began to suffer from mental illness, heart disease, arthritis and glandular problems. Zaret confirmed he had also developed a microwave cataract and warned that his other diseases could 'be related at least on a contributory basis to microwave exposure'.[26]

■Joseph Towne, a retired US air force radar technician, developed cataracts after working with a new radar system. The air force told him the cataracts were due to diabetes – a disease he did not have. Zaret diagnosed microwaves as their cause.[27]

■Abnormal cancer rates have been found in Rutherford, New Jersey, a town with some 6,400 sources of microwaves. 5 children at the local primary school developed cancer – the odds against which are estimated to be 10 million to 1. After measuring the intensity of microwaves in the area, the National Bureau of Standards warned that the 'field strengths are high enough to imply something'.[28]

■The number of cases of cancer and heart attacks increased in the North Karelia region of Finland after a large Soviet radar station went into operation just across the Russo-Finnish border.[29]

■In 1981, in a landmark decision, New York State's Workers' Compensation Board ruled that Stephen Yannon, a radio technician who had worked with microwaves for 15 years before his death in 1974, had died of chronic exposure to microwave radiation. Yannon, who tuned television transmitters, had been subjected while working to microwave levels of just 1.2 milliwatts per square centimetre – well within the 10 milliwatt standard. 'After (working) eleven years, Yannon began visiting doctors with complaints of problems in sight and hearing', reports Keith Hindley of the *Sunday Times.* 'He eventually developed cataracts, a loss of balance and severe premature senility. His mental state deteriorated so badly that he recognised no-one and wasted away physically, losing 8 stone in weight. When he died, his withered crooked frame weighed just under 5 stone. His employers had claimed that he died of Alheimer's disease – an ailment of old age which is common enough for one person in ten over 60 to have it – but few doctors agreed.'[30] Publicity given to the Yannon case prompted a furore in Britain where the Post Office Engineering Union accused the government of not sponsoring enough research on microwaves and microwave standards. The National Radiological Protection Board promised to publish a new set of safety standards in 1982.[31]

But the real bombshell came when the Russian bombardment of the American embassy in Moscow was finally made public. Newspaper columnist, Jack Anderson, had broken the story in 1972 but it was not until 1976 that the problem was officially recognised. Blood tests on embassy staff revealed counts of lymphocytes – the white blood cells which counter infection – were 40 per cent higher than those amongst foreign service employees serving in other countries.[32] Such high lymphocyte counts are frequently associated with cancer and, significantly, the US ambassador, Walter Stoessel, later resigned because he was suffering from a rare blood disorder resembling leukemia.[33] Two of his predecessors had died of cancer and three embassy children were flown home to the United States to be treated for blood disorders of an unspecified nature.[34] But most disturbing of all, chromosome changes had been found in the blood of four embassy officials.[35] Indeed, a 1969 Pentagon report – kept hidden from the public for ten years – had warned that '43 per cent of the subjects exposed to the Moscow embassy irradiation should be classified as . . . having actually experienced high risk of mutagenic exposure'.[36] It also emerged that there was an unusually high rate of deformed babies born to women working at the embassy.[37]

For its part, the State Department (which had classified the Moscow embassy as an 'unhealthful post' and given all employees a 20 per cent pay rise) issued a flurry of denials that there was any connection between the diseases diagnosed in embassy staff and their exposure to microwaves.[38] In its defence, it cited a top-secret study performed in the sixties and known as Project Pandora which it is claimed had shown no biological effects from exposure to low-intensity microwaves. It was impossible to verify that claim, however, for the Pentagon had destroyed all the data on which the study was based.[39]

Paul Brodeur believes that behind the State Department's worried denials lies 'the deeper conviction in high government circles that the radiation to which tens of thousands of civilian and military personnel have been subjected has inflicted genetic damage upon them'.[40] He points out that it has been known for nearly two decades that low levels of microwave radiation can cause chromosomal abnormalities in the roots of garlic and genetic mutations in the cells of animals and insects similar to those produced by ionising radiation.[41] Then, in 1964, scientists at Johns Hopkins University linked Down's syndrome – the fatal chromosome break which causes mongolism – to the exposure of fathers to radar.[42]

The best documented evidence of genetic damage to humans from exposure to microwaves comes from a study of birth defects in Alabama, where the US army has a large helicopter training base at Fort Rucker, Dale County. Within thirty miles of the base, there are forty-six radar installations. Dr Peter Peacock, Professor of Public Health and Epidemiology at the University of Alabama, discovered that between July 1969 and November 1970, there had been a significant increase in the incidence of certain birth defects in 7 out of Alabama's 67 counties.[43]

'Peacock found that during the seventeen-month period, 17 white children suffering from congenital clubfoot had been delivered in two particular counties, Dale and Coffee. The expected number of children with this affliction had been less than 4,' writes Paul Brodeur. 'They also learned that the rate of children born with congenital abnormalities of the heart was significantly higher in Dale County than in other parts of Alabama.' All seventeen children had been delivered at the Lister Army Hospital, Fort Rucker, and all were the children of helicopter pilots who, because they fly at low altitudes, are exposed to radar waves for most of their working lives. [44]

Although Peacock was at pains to point out that these findings did not establish conclusive proof of a connection between congenital malformations and exposure to radar, the army immediately began to block further research into the problem. It refused to release medical files on its pilots and repeatedly turned down proposals by Peacock for a follow-up study. Nor were the air force and navy any more helpful. Any study, they claimed, would be meaningless unless they released the radar levels to which pilots were exposed. And those levels were a military secret. [45]

But by now, however, the 10 milliwatt standard was under attack from another quarter – one over which the military had far less control. Not that it did not try to silence the furore that ensued.

Until twenty years ago, the standard view of biologists was that life was to be understood entirely through chemistry. That view was first challenged by Albert Szent-Gyorgyi, the Nobel Prize laureate who isolated Vitamin D and who was also at the forefront of the research which led to the discovery of the Krebs cycle. In the early sixties, Szent-Gyorgyi postulated that the development of cancer could not be explained by chemistry alone and that subtle changes in the electrical fields within cells must also be taken into account. That theory was dismissed almost out of hand by the bulk of the American scientific establishment and despite his considerable scientific reputation, Szent-Gyorgyi was unable to obtain funds to follow up his ideas. [46]

Szent-Gyorgyi's work prompted Robert Becker, an orthopaedic surgeon at the Veterans Administration Hospital in Syracuse, New York, to research into the electrical – or solid state – properties of biological tissues and, in particular, into the effects of electrical fields of the bone-healing mechanism of the human body. He found that the healing process could be accelerated if an injured limb was placed in a small electrical field. But whereas the electrical field was beneficial to broken bones, Becker found that unbroken bones developed tumours. [47] Meanwhile, a further research programme headed by

Becker's colleague, Andrew Marino, was starting to look into the possible side effects of electrical fields on animals. In a series of experiments, Marino, a biophysicist, had found that rats exposed to electrical fields comparable in strength to those produced at ground level by a 750 kilovolt power line were severely stunted; that blood steroid levels were decreased; and that there was a dramatic rise in infant mortality.[48] The rats also showed symptoms consistent with chronic stress. Becker and Marino concluded that the electrical field affected the central nervous system and activated a stress-response mechanism which could in theory produce a wide range of diseases and pathological conditions.[49] Subsequent research (this time on mice) has provided equally damning evidence. Subjected to vertical electrical fields, the mice not only lost weight but like the rats showed increased rates of infant mortality.[50]

Becker and Marino are now convinced that low-frequency electromagnetic fields can affect both animals and man and suggest that the mechanism lies in their ability to 'trigger' biological responses. It has been known for some time that small electrical currents within the body play a vital role in controlling biological activities. 'Cells in the body exist in equilibrium with their immediate electrical microenvironment,' says Marino. 'Certain changes in this microenvironment result in information being transmitted to cells which is capable of controlling their function. Thus a given cell may be triggered to differentiate or build bone or increase protein synthesis or decrease hormone output.'[51] Because these electrical charges convey information – the cells themselves providing the energy for a process to occur – even a small outside electrical stimulus could produce a biological effect.

Indeed, many scientists now privately express fears that the body's natural electrical currents may play such a vital role in cell differentiation that by presenting abnormal signals to the cells, low-frequency electromagnetic radiation could cause long-term genetic damage. Already experiments have shown that cell division is disrupted in mice subjected to electrical fields of 50 hertz – a frequency equivalent to that beneath a high-voltage wire.[52] Indeed, so little is known about the body's natural use of electricity that, in Becker's view, 'the chronic exposure of humans to electrical fields should be viewed as human experimentation'.[53]

That view is apparently endorsed by the Soviet authorities. 'In 1962, after the first 500 kilovolt lines had been operating in the Soviet Union for several months,' reports Louise Young, whose book *Power Over People* did much to bring the health hazards of overhead electric cables to light, 'men working at the substations began to complain of headaches and a general feeling of malaise.'[54, 55] Other workers complained of abnormal fatigue, sleepiness and decreased sexual vigour – symptoms they associated with exposure to electrical fields.

A long-term study of these effects was undertaken. The investigators concluded that work at 500 and 750 kilovolt substations without protective measures resulted in 'shattering the dynamic state of the central nervous system, the heart and blood vessel system and in changing blood structure'.[56] That initial finding has subsequently been confirmed in over one hundred reports published in the Soviet Union. Other effects have also been documented: mice exposed to magnetic fields of 50 hertz quickly lose their ability to expel foreign matter from the liver, spleen and lungs; the function of the glands of rats exposed to fields of similar intensity is grossly impaired; and a survey of some two hundred workers at 220, 330 and 500 kilovolt substations has shown a significant increase in the haemoglobin content of their blood.[57] Russian scientists now believe that electrical fields as low as 50 volts per centimetre can have an adverse effect on human health.[58]

As a result of these findings, the Soviet authorities have imposed strict rules relating to the exposure of electricity workers and the general public to electrical fields of more than 250 volts/cm, and even in fields of 200/cm unprotected workers may only be exposed for ten minutes in any 24-hour period. A 360-foot zone centred on the line is restricted to certain authorised personnel; it may not be used for recreation; buildings, bus shelters and other places where people may congregate are forbidden in the area; no vehicle is allowed to stop or be refuelled under the line – for fear of a spark igniting its fuel – and if a vehicle does break down it must be towed away before any repairs are done; and finally, metal shields must be used over the seats of farm machinery.[59]

Both Becker and Marino knew of those Soviet standards before they became involved in the controversy over the effects of low-frequency radiation. But, ironically, it was an American study which embroiled them in their biggest battle. In September 1973, they presented the results of their research on rats to a meeting of the New

York Academy of Sciences. After the meeting they were approached by a Captain Paul Tyler, a US navy officer, who invited Becker to sit on the navy's Ad Hoc Committee for the Review of Biomedical and Ecological Effects of Extremely Low-Frequency (ELF) Radiation. The navy, Tyler explained, was building a massive radar antenna which would allow submarines to communicate even when they were submerged to a depth of 4,000 feet. Code-named Project Sanguine, the antenna consisted of a grid of wires buried over 25,000 square miles of Northern Wisconsin and under new environmental laws the navy was required to submit studies on the possible impact of Sanguine's ELF fields. [60]

Becker accepted Tyler's offer and in December 1973, the committee sat to review the scientific literature on the health hazards of ELF radiation. Its report was hardly reassuring. In particular, the committee's members expressed unanimous concern over the initial results of a contemporary study which showed that electrical fields of the same strength as Sanguine's could cause a rise in the levels of serum triglycerides in human blood – an effect linked to the incidence of heart attacks. The implication of that and other studies revealing that those living near Sanguine were likely to suffer mental illness and other behavioural effects was not lost on the committee, for the electrical fields created by Sanguine were *one million* times less intense than those under high voltage power lines. [61] Indeed, the committee was sufficiently alarmed to recommend that the US government 'be apprised of (these) positive findings and the possible significance should they be validated . . . to the large population at risk in the United States who are exposed to 60 hertz fields from power lines and other hertz sources'. [62] No action was taken and the report was buried by the navy for two years.

The concerns expressed by the committee were very much in Becker's mind, however, when he returned to Syracuse after attending the December meeting of the committee in Washington. He had scarcely had time to pour himself a drink when he read in the local newspaper that plans were afoot to build a 765 kilovolt high voltage line from the Canadian border to a substation near Utica, upstate New York. Not surprisingly, he wrote to the Chairman of the New York Public Services Commission (PSC) – the body which oversees planning permission for such projects – warning of the committee's findings and recommending that the PSC obtain a copy of its report.[63] As a result, both he and Marino were invited to testify before preliminary hearings on the desirability of the proposed line.[64]

'Very shortly after we both testified,' recalls Marino, 'the tone of the hearing changed dramatically. What had begun as a proceeding involving two small upstate New York utility companies, quickly took on a much wider focus. We viewed our testimony as a contribution towards the development of better, safe high voltage transmission lines. Soon after it was released, however, reports began to circulate that Rochester Gas and Electric – one of the companies involved – would reject our testimony in its entirety. Public comments from the Power Authority of the State of New York (PASNY) quickly revealed that it, too, would oppose as unnecessary any attempts to protect the public from exposure to the fields of its proposed line . . . a siege mentality developed almost overnight, with the various New York utility companies united in opposition to the ideas that chronic exposure to the fields of high voltage transmission lines should be prevented because of the potential health hazard. There was a yet more ominous development. One could easily perceive a possible community of interests between the utilities and the navy, which still sought permission to build Sanguine. Given the commitment to Sanguine, it was predictable that the navy would employ its resources to oppose a judgement by the Public Service Commission that exposure to transmission line fields was a health hazard.'[65]

The possibility of a link between the navy and the electricity companies appeared still stronger when the companies announced their choice of expert witnesses. The names read like a roll call of Department of Defense scientists: Solomon Michaelson, a DOD-funded researcher; Edwin Carstensen and Morton Miller, both well known for their view that ELF radiation could not cause biological damage; and Herman Schwan, a consultant to the navy and the architect of the 10 milliwatt standard for microwave exposure.[66]

Meanwhile, the navy's attempts to suppress research which challenged the received widsom of low-frequency radiation were becoming increasingly obvious. Indeed, in his testimony, Marino told the Public Services Commission:

'In early 1975, the navy published a compilation of some of the

ELF research that had been revealed to the Ad Hoc Committee in December 1973. The document described two kinds of research projects. The first type of ELF research was performed in-house at a navy research facility by navy personnel; the second type was performed at universities by faculty personnel. With two exceptions, the in-house navy projects all concluded that ELF fields didn't cause any biological effects. Most of the studies by the university scientists, however, found positive effects due to ELF fields. By the end of 1975, the university scientists who had reported ELF bioeffects had lost their navy research funding, and the head of the Naval Aerospace Medical Research Laboratory (NARML), whose research team was responsible for the two exceptions regarding in-house navy research, had retired. The scientist, Dr Dietrich Beischer, had an international reputation in the area of biological effects of magnetic fields. Beischer has been in seclusion and he has not written or spoken publicly since his retirement.

'Some navy in-house research projects just disappeared . . . Perhaps the most serious instance occurred in connection with an ELF research project at the Naval Air Development Centre at Warminster, Pennsylvania. Around 1971, an ELF bioeffects team was founded by the navy at Warminster. A number of different kinds of experiment were performed; by 1975, it was clear that the most important were those involving thirty-day exposure of rats. The scientists exposed the rats to a range of very weak ELF electric fields. Although the details of the experiments remained secret until 1976, the experimental procedure and the results observed were remarkably similar to the experiments performed by Dr Becker and myself in 1975, except that the navy research team employed weak, Sanguine-strength electric fields. The navy scientists consistently found that the exposed rats were stunted. The navy Sanguine officials, however, felt that the results must be flawed because they were not "consistent"; the navy scientists observed stunting at all field strengths studied, while the navy Sanguine officials believed that if the effects were real it would have to be proportional to dose, resulting in more stunting at higher field strengths. The navy Sanguine officials made several trips to the Warminster facility in an attempt to find a defect in the experimental set-up. They found none, however, and the scientists continued to report stunting of growth, whereupon the navy terminated the project and dissolved the research team. The various periodic reports which the group had filed with the navy Sanguine officials were not released.

'In 1975 and thereafter, the only substantial ELF research conducted by the navy was work aimed at undoing the in-house positive results reported in previous years.'[67]

Embarrassed by such revelations, the navy announced in 1976 that it intended to conduct another study on the effects of Project Sanguine.[68]

That study was to be carried out under the aegis of the National Academy of Sciences and chaired by Woodland Hastings, professor of biology at Harvard. On 13 January 1976, Hastings wrote to Marino asking him to participate in the study as a consultant. Before accepting, Marino inquired who else was sitting on the committee and was told that its members had almost all been selected by the navy. Among them were Schwan, Michaelson and Miller.

Marino was amazed. All three men had just completed their testimony before the Public Service Commission where they had adamantly denied that the fields around high-voltage transmission lines could cause biological harm. If they considered fields one million times stronger than Sanguine's to be harmless, how likely was it that they would find the weaker fields dangerous? Would not the study be prejudiced from the start? When Hastings heard this, he allegedly told Marino that he would resign his chairmanship unless the three men were stripped of their membership of the committee. He also promised to check the 'bias forms' – questionnaires designed to reveal any conflict of interests – which had been completed by Schwan, Michaelson and Miller when they were accepted on to the committee. The next day, he telephoned Marino and revealed that all three men had failed to disclose either their close ties with electrical companies or their previous public statements about ELF health standards.[69] Nonetheless, they remained on the committee. And two years later, after a mysterious change of heart, Hastings was to tell Susan Schiefelbein of the *Saturday Review* that Marino was 'a quack' and that his testimony at the Public Service Commission hearings had been thrown out of court as 'evasive and deceitful'.[70]

That accusation rested on comments made by judges Thomas

Matias and Harold Colbeth during the PSC hearings. In their Recommended Decision to the Public Service Commission, they accused Marino of being 'reckless and inaccurate in his public statements' and 'evasive and argumentative under cross-examination'.[71] Apparently, those criticisms failed to persuade the PSC, however, for in its final judgement it not only exonerated Marino but also ordered the electricity companies to set up a fund to research further the effects of ELF radiation.[72] Indeed, the PSC acknowledged that 'although the record before us is in many ways reassuring – it does not show that the electrical and magnetic fields of the lines as proposed will induce effects endangering human health and safety – it contains unrefuted inferences of possible risks that we cannot responsibly ignore'[73]

But perhaps most intriguing, letters obtained under the Freedom of Information Act reveal that Judge Colbeth had written to Asher Sheppard, a researcher working at the Brain Research Institute at the University of California, asking him to 'furnish assistance in evaluating conflicting testimonies'. Sheppard had been paid $5,224 for his services and was told by Colbeth that it was hoped that his report could be put 'bodily into our decision with a few language changes for consistency of style'. At the time Sheppard, who once worked for Con Edison, was a consultant to the American Electric Power Company. Indeed, he was writing a report for them. Its subject: the biological effects of extremely low-frequency radiation.[74]

Across the Atlantic, a similar controversy was raging. Nestling in the Charmouth Valley lies the small hamlet of Fishpond, Dorset. Fifty years ago the post-impressionist painter, Pissarro, had come there to paint its sweeping landscapes now irrevocably ruined by huge pylons which straddle the ten or so houses in the hamlet. Those living under the pylons complain of chronic headaches, eye-strain, blackouts, exhaustion, depression and even blood-cell disorders.

Fishpond's plight has been brought to the public's attention largely through the efforts of one extremely tenacious woman, Mrs Hilary Bacon. Since 1973, when she moved into her present cottage, a converted chapel, she has been engaged in a running battle with the Central Electricity Generating Board (CEGB) whose reluctance to part with information has only been matched by her own determination to unearth it.

'It was early spring when I experienced my first blackout,' recalls Bacon. 'I had gone out to cut some broccoli from my vegetable garden which is right underneath the pylons. Suddenly, there was what I can only describe as a "black light" everywhere: I could still see but I became totally disorientated.'[75] Later, Bacon discovered that several other villagers had suffered the same experience: indeed, her son, Guy, had blacked out whilst riding his motorbike beneath the wires. Two or three weeks earlier, the CEGB had increased the voltage going through the transmission lines – but no one in Fishpond had been told.[76]

It was an article in the *Listener* that first alerted Bacon to the possibility that the blackouts and headaches afflicting Fishpond might be connected to the electricity lines over the village. The article reported that a preponderance of positive ions in the atmosphere was linked to depression – and that electricity lines created such ions. As a result, Bacon wrote to the author of the article and before long was in touch with the Institute of Industrial Health. There she found an impressive library of reports from Italy, Russia and America on the effects of low-frequency radiation, but when she produced that evidence at a meeting with the CEGB the board dismissed it out of hand.[77]

The opportunity to pin the CEGB down in public, forcing it to justify its assurances that power lines have no important biological effects, came about by an extraordinary chance. Partly due to the ill effects of the pylons on their health, two of Hilary Bacon's closest friends, Eustace and Kathleen Yeomans, moved from Fishpond to Innsworth, Gloucester, only to learn a year later that plans were afoot to reroute a nearby section of a 400 kilovolt supergrid so that it would now run closer to Innsworth. They also heard that the CEGB were intending to increase the capacity of the power lines in order to take electricity from four nuclear power stations that it is planning to build in the area in the late 1980s. A public inquiry was called in October 1978 to hear objections to the scheme, and local residents, through the Yeomans, invited Hilary Bacon to testify on their behalf.

The determination of the villagers of Innsworth to raise the issue of health hazards was, in part, inspired by Marino's testimony at the New York Public Service Commission hearings. Like Marino, they presented studies from the Soviet Union warning of the health hazards of non-ionising radiation and outlining the precautions taken to protect Russian workers and civilians. By comparison, they argued, the measures taken to reduce risks under power lines in Britain and the USA are derisory. Refusing to admit any health hazards, the only precautions taken by the CEGB is to warn farmers not to stack crops or use ladders and tall equipment near overhead lines and not to place electric fences beneath or parallel to the wires.

Indeed, the CEGB rejects the Russian evdidence out of hand. It maintains that it is not objective; that it lacks sufficient data and precise clinical diagnosis; that the reports are couched in vague terms and cannot be taken as incontrovertible evidence; that the scientific methods used by the Soviets are less sound than those used in the West; that no-one knows the basis on which the Soviet standards are set; and finally that other research refutes the evidence in the Russian studies. [78] It is worth noting that precisely the same reaction was shown by Western scientists when the Russians first produced evidence on the low-level effects of ionising radiation.* [79]

Given the importance of the Soviet studies to the debate, one might have expected the CEGB to use the Innsworth inquiry as an opportunity to rebut the Russian evidence in detail. It did not do so,

---

* Far from the Russian evidence being scant, it is the philosophy behind British and American safety standards that appears to be lacking. Dr Karel Marha, the professor at the Institute of Industrial Hygiene and Occupational Disease in Prague, put her finger on it when she remarked – in respect of microwave radiation – that Eastern European standards are set 'not only to avoid damage but also to avoid discomfiture in people'.

American and British objections to the Russian studies might be on firmer ground if proper health surveys had been carried out on workers in their own electrical industries. Thus until 1978 the only US study to have been carried out was based on a very small and inadequate investigation undertaken at Johns Hopkins University and financed by a major electrical utility, The American Electric Power Company. 'Starting in 1963, eleven linesmen were given medical examinations over a nine-year period,' reports Louise Young. 'No control group was used; no quantitative data was reported on the length of time and level of exposure experienced by these men; and no clinical information was reported. During the nine years, one man dropped out of the study (because he quit his job) and eight of the others became supervisors. At the end of the report, a general statement was made that no sigificant changes of any kind were found as a result of general physical examinations. Three of the men did have apparently low sperm counts in the last examination, but the counts had been quite varied throughout the nine years and therefore it was concluded that "it would be hazardous to draw any conclusions from such a small sample. Indeed, the small number of men studied is the most serious flaw of the whole experiment." '

however. Indeed, in his evidence to the inquiry, Dr John Bonnell, the CEGB's Deputy Chief Nuclear Health and Safety Officer and one of the Board's principal witnesses, cited only four of the Russian papers relevant to the issue at hand – this at a time when the Soviet literature contained several hundred studies on the biological effects of exposure to the types of electrical fields under consideration.[80, 81] The studies cited by Bonnell dated back to the mid-1960s and early 1970s and involved linesmen, switchyard operators and 'groups of volunteers deliberately exposed to high voltage fields'.[82] All showed biological effects.[83]

Nonetheless, stated Bonnell, the studies could be criticised on several grounds: in one case, 'The symptoms described by the Russians were entirely subjective and for the most part vague and non-specific, and in general terms could be related to the degree of motivation of the workmen themselves.' In another case, the experimental tests employed were 'Not described in detail and direct attempts to obtain such detailed information from the authors (had) not been successful.'[84] As for the final study quoted, said Bonnell, the scientific procedures used in the experiments were 'Open to very serious criticism'.[85] Moreover, he claimed: 'Investigations in Western European countries, the USA and Canada over prolonged periods of time have not confirmed Russian findings. In fact, in all cases negative results were reported from studies of the health of exposed linesmen, switchyard operators, farmers working under high voltage lines and experiments on human volunteers.'[86] To support that claim, Bonnell cited three references.[87] He went on to quote another five studies which had found no adverse health effects amongst those exposed to electrical fields of the relevant strength.[88] All but one of those studies involved electrical workers or human volunteers exposed for short periods of time (in one case 'up to three hours').[89] The exception was an epidemiological study comparing the health of those living within twenty-five metres of a 200-400 kilovolt line with the health of those living more than 125 metres from the line.[90] Those involved in that study were employees of Electricité de France and their families.[91] EDF is the French equivalent of the CEGB.

However, it is a moot point whether the studies Bonnell did cite (those examining the health of linesmen, sub-station workers and volunteers) were really relevant to the issue at hand. As Martin Weitz reported in *New Statesman*: 'The experience of workers exposed to high voltage electric fields may have no bearing on individuals who are continuously exposed day and night seven days a week to levels of electrical pollution which could be between 40 and 1000 times higher than occurs naturally.'[92]

The CEGB, however, denied that such high levels could be reached under high-voltage lines. They argued that tests they had done at Fishpond – before the voltage of the lines was increased – showed that the strengths of the electrical field at ground level measured only 6000 volts per metre – well within the Russian safety limits but sufficient to light up a fluorescent tube.[93, 94]

That measurement, however, is highly misleading: Dr David Smith told the Innsworth inquiry that in reality levels as high as 120,000 volts per metre could be reached at Fishpond.[95] The reason, he said, was that any object placed under a power line – from a pram to a person – tends to concentrate the electrical field, thus enhancing it greatly.[96] In effect, the electrical field itself need not be very high for high voltages to be experienced.[97]

Nor is that the only example of the CEGB trying to allay fears by quoting inadequate – and often irrelevant – measurements. For a long time it has been known that positive and negative ions – electrically charged particles – are formed around the high voltage wires and that the preponderance of positive ions in the atmosphere is associated with a cluster of health risks from behavioural changes to a general feeling of malaise. Half way through the Innsworth inquiry, the CEGB learned that Dr Leslie Hawkins of the University of Surrey was going to measure the concentration of ions around Fishpond. 'When the CEGB discovered (this)', reports Martin Weitz, 'they got worried and thought that his readings might be used against them at the inquiry. In fact there was never any intention to do so because, to make any sensible interpretation, ion measurements need to be taken over a long period of time and in varying climatic conditions. This however did not deter the CEGB borrowing an ion measuring device and spending a day taking totally meaningless measurements under power lines in Surrey and inside one of their employee's kitchens. These measurements were then presented at the inquiry as evidence that power lines do not produce unusual amounts of ionisation.'[98]

Significantly, the CEGB's measurements were taken on a particularly calm day when the chances were high that the positive and negative ions around the wires will recombine – thereby neutralising each other – before they reach the ground.[99] Dr Hawkins suggests that under windier conditions this recombination would not occur, particularly if the earth's natural electrical field were strong in the area.[100] In any event, a measurement taken on one day at a different location hardly supplies convincing proof that ionisation around the power lines at Fishpond is inconsequential.

Since the Innsworth inquiry, Dr Hawkins has been trying to find funds in order to conduct a long-term survey of ionisation at Fishpond and elsewhere. Although he was at one point offered £10,000 by the Health and Safety Executive to undertake such a survey, that offer was subsequently withdrawn apparently on the advice of the National Radiological Board.[101]

In the course of the Innsworth inquiry, Bacon and others pointed to numerous studies cited by Marino in his evidence to the New York Public Service Commission. Although in his proof of evidence, Dr Bonnell did not deal with those studies, he did mention the work of Dr Becker and Dr Marino and the conclusions they had reached. He did not, however, rebut their evidence through an analysis of their experiments. Instead, he told the inspectors: 'In their assessment of Dr Marino's testimony, the Administrative Law Judges Mathias and Colbeth discounted his evidence on the grounds that "Dr Marino's experimental work was not conducted carefully enough for the results to be believable." They further commented that "the indications of careless procedures, faulty statistics and unsupported extrapolations from his own experiments make it impossible to place any substantial reliance on Dr Marino's scientific research as set forth in this record." ' Bonnell went on to add: 'I think it is relevant that the judges make the following observation, "Dr Marino at times appeared to be more interested in the personalities of his adversaries than he was in scientific method or theory. Unfortunately the impression sometimes created was not of a scientist objectively pursuing his craft." '[102]

Taken by themselves, these comments of Mathias and Colbeth are, of course, a devastating indictment of Marino's work. But, as we have seen, the Public Service Commission of the State of New York overruled the assessment of the two administrative law judges and in fact exonerated Marino. Bonnell did not mention that ruling, however, in his proof of evidence. Nor did he tell the inspectors that the staff of the Public Service Commission had told the New York hearings that, in its opinion, Marino's work on mice (unlike his work on rats which they criticised) consisted of 'well controlled and well designed experiments with no major flaws' which 'withstood every criticism levelled at them'.[103] Nor did Bonnell mention that, in its final ruling, the Public Service Commission had noted: 'Staff also take the position that its witness Marino's credibility cannot be used as the basis for deciding the issue and that the applicant's vigorous efforts to discredit him were more suitable to a slander trial than a fact-finding scientific investigation.'[104] Small wonder, perhaps, that Mr Patrick Clarkson, the barrister for the objectors at Innsworth, described Bonnell's evidence as 'selective' and commented: 'Anything that is contrary to his views is dismissed as irrelevant.'[105]

But if Bonnell's original proof of evidence proved somewhat controversial, his subsequent rebuttal testimony sparked a furore which has still not abated. In his evidence to the inquiry, Bonnell had stated that animal experiments at Battelle North West Laboratories in Portland, Oregon, had confirmed earlier research which showed animals exposed to low-frequency electrical fields did not suffer ill effects.[106] Under cross-examination, Bonnell said he would send for the Battelle study because it strengthened his case. However, in his earlier testimony Bonnell had told the inspectors that animal experiments were notoriously unreliable for assessing human hazards.[107]

The matter did not rest there, however. After the objectors at the inquiry had been examined, the CEGB's barrister asked permission from the inspectors to present 'rebuttal testimony' – a request that surprised Patrick Clarkson.[108] Nonetheless, permission was granted and Bonnell once again took the witness stand. But if anyone at the inquiry was expecting him to present the new Battelle research, they were to be disappointed. He did not mention it. Indeed, it was ultimately to be used by Clarkson in his summing up for the objectors for, by and large, it *endorsed* the findings of Marino and others.*[109]

---

* The objectors were quick to point out that if the Battelle findings had been negative, they would have proved very little. In fact, there is no contradiction between some researchers finding positive effects from low-frequency electrical fields and others finding none. Negative findings do not vindicate the position of those who claim that the hazards are non-existent; they simply show that, under

Instead of presenting new scientific evidence, Bonnell proceeded to 'diagnose' Hilary Bacon's medical and psychological condition, making repeated reference to her age and the fact that she was divorced.[110] That 'diagnosis' was made without reference to Bacon's medical record to which Bonnell did not have access. For his part Bonnell claims that Bacon refused him such access. Bacon, however, denies that allegation and told her lawyer that she was quite willing to give Bonnell her medical record provided that he also requested the medical files of those other villagers in Fishpond who (in a sworn deposition) had stated that they also suffered from the symptoms she described.

Quite why Bonnell chose to discuss Hilary Bacon's medical condition in his rebuttal testimony is somewhat unclear. In 1981, in an article in the *Guardian*, Bacon alleged it was because Bonnell wished to discredit her evidence by making her out to be a neurotic, whose symptoms were psychosomatic.[111] The article brought an immediate threat of a libel suit from Bonnell and the *Guardian* published a suitable apology. The story does not end there, however, for Bacon and Bonnell were to cross swords again in the summer of 1982.

The occasion was another inquiry, held at Haddington in East Lothian, Scotland. The inquiry had been set up to consider a proposed high-voltage transmission line from Torness, where a nuclear power station is under construction, across South-East Scotland to Edinburgh and Glasgow. Bacon had been asked to testify on behalf of a local resident and Bonnell was appearing for the South of Scotland Electricity Board (a quite separate body from the CEGB). Before giving evidence, Bacon submitted her proof of evidence to all the parties concerned. Immediately before Bonnell was

---

certain conditions, electrical fields will not induce biological effects. As Marino put it to the New York inquiry: 'A whole range of different interactions are possible between transmission line fields, people and the environment. They vary from a brief encounter to chronic exposure such as occurs for individuals living very close to the transmission line. The lesson of the literature is that some situations will probably result in biological effects, and others will probably not . . . Obviously both conclusions can be true simultaneously, and the truth of one does not imply the falsity of the other.' Yet if positive results are found, the warning lights should begin to flash, for however inadequate animal experiments might be, they are the only advance indication we have of possible dangers to human health from our various activities. To ignore them is both intellectually dishonest – and foolhardy.

due to testify, the barrister for the SSEB demanded that certain portions of Bacon's evidence be retracted. The offending sections, she learnt, referred to her interpretation of Bonnell's rebuttal testimony at Innsworth. If she repeated her allegations, she was told, she could run the risk of a libel action.[112] 'The threat of a libel suit frightened me,' Bacon recalls. 'But I don't like being bullied, so I decided not to retract the offending passages but rather to rewrite them in more detail.'

Bacon's testimony at Haddington showed her to be no slouch when it came to doing her homework. In his evidence to the inquiry, Bonnell had stated that no less an authority than the prestigious *British Medical Journal* had reassured its readers that high-voltage power lines posed no threat to human health.[113] This indeed was true. In October 1980, a doctor had written to the *Journal* stating that a patient had complained of feeling unwell, with a range of vague symptoms such as tiredness, blurred vision, paraesthesia, vertigo and feeling depressed, which he (attributed) to living beneath high tension electricity cables. Was there any evidence, the doctor asked, that such cables were a health hazard?[114]

Underneath the doctor's letter, the *BMJ* printed the reply of an anonymous expert:

'The growth in the demand for electricity over the years has led to the use of high transmission voltages: 225 kilovolts has been used for over 40 years and 400 kilovolts for the past 20. Lately the regional office of the World Health Organisation has reviewed works on the effects on man. The organisation held a meeting in West Germany of experts in electropathology and radiation from most industrially developed countries. After making a critical study of the physical and physiological phenomena occurring when a living organism is placed in an electric field, and reviewing publications on the subject, these authors concluded that electric fields were harmless up to transmission voltages of 400 kilovolts. On the basis of current available results for extra high voltage transmission lines, they considered that these conclusions could be extrapolated to transmission voltages of up to 800 kilovolts. It would seem, therefore, that other clinical causes should be sought for the patient's symptoms.'

However, it was not disclosed at the inquiry that Dr Bonnell was a co-author of the only study cited by the anonymous reviewer.[115] More damning still, Hilary Bacon produced evidence that the anonymous reviewer was none other than a Dr R.H.P. Fernandez, Senior Medical Officer for the CEGB and a close colleague of Bonnell. That evidence emerged as a result of a correspondence between a doctor friendly to Hilary Bacon and the *BMJ*. In September 1981, that doctor had written to the *BMJ* asking for the name of the GP who had originally written describing the symptoms of the patient who lived under the power lines. The *BMJ* had written back saying that it was their policy 'never to divulge the name of our experts without their permission'.[116] In fact, that information had not been requested. Nonetheless, the *BMJ* promised to forward the doctor's letter to the 'expert concerned'. Two weeks later, the doctor received the following reply from Fernandez:

'The *British Medical Journal* have been in contact with me regarding your interest in my answer to a question in the *BMJ* on October 25 1980. If I can be of help in any way, please do contact me and certainly I am sure that any help my employer, the Generating Board, can give technically will be given. It may be best that you would like to have a word with me or indeed Dr J.A. Bonnell who is involved with me in work on this subject.'[117]

It is, perhaps, interesting to note that when both Hilary Bacon and her local GP wrote to the *BMJ* they were told that it was not the *BMJ*'s policy to reveal the names of their experts.[118]

Shortly after testifying at Haddington, Hilary Bacon had a serious car accident which nearly resulted in the loss of her eyesight. Driving to fetch her son from Taunton, she blacked out and crashed her car into the side of a stone bridge. That blackout was the third she had experienced in one year.[119] Although it has not been proven, it is possible that such blackouts could be caused by the type of low-level magnetic fields normally associated with high voltage cables. Dr Cyril Smith, of Salford University, for instance, has shown that the current beneath high voltage power lines is sufficient to produce natural pain killers, known as endorphins, in the brain.[120] Those endorphins create a feeling of euphoria. 'But doctors have found that, like man-made opiates, they can be addictive,' reports Andrew Veitch in the *Guardian*. 'The electromagnetic field beneath power lines can fluctuate from hour to hour – it can vary by a factor of ten according to the CEGB. So, Dr Smith suggests, when the current is at the critical endorphin-producing level, the person beneath the power line feels fine. When it drops beneath that level, the person experiences withdrawal symptoms.'[121] Was that what Hilary Bacon experienced when she had her car crash? Or did she suffer a form of epileptic attack – an effect which at least one researcher has found to persist in animals even after they are withdrawn from an electric field?[122]

At the time of writing, the results of the Haddington inquiry are not known.[123] Those of the Innsworth inquiry, however, were published in 1980.[124] After considering the inspectors' report, the Secretary of State for Energy deemed that there was insufficient evidence to support the view that exposure to electromagnetic fields was harmful to health. Nevertheless, the CEGB was 'required' by the Secretary of State to report annually on its monitoring of the literature on the biological effects of the ELF fields; to conduct its own research on the subject; and to conduct a programme on ion measurements.[125]

To date, the CEGB has produced just one report – on the effect of overhead lines on pacemakers (it was concluded that the latest type of pacemaker, which is not yet available, would not be affected). To my knowledge no study has yet been published on the health effects of magnetic fields, nor of electric fields, nor of the two combined.[126] However, the CEGB is carrying out a survey of the psychological effects of living in electromagnetic fields three times the strength of those experienced under high voltage wires.[127] Dr Cyril Smith has argued that such high levels may not in fact be as biologically harmful as lower, fluctuating fields.[128] To judge from a letter from David Mellor, Parliamentary Under Secretary of State for the Department of Energy, to Jim Spicer, the MP for Hilary Bacon's constituency, it would appear that it will be some time before any study on the biological effects of overhead high-voltage lines is forthcoming from the CEGB: as he puts it, 'Research of this nature is bound to take some time before it is possible to come to final conclusions on the matter.'[129]

Meanwhile the evidence that electromagnetic fields of low intensity (and even magnetic fields by themselves) can cause biological damage continues to mount.[130] And whilst the CEGB waits for 'final conclusions', the inhabitants of Fishpond and elsewhere also wait, living daily with symptoms that the CEGB would no doubt prefer to describe as 'psychosomatic'. 'When it's a very misty day you feel, oh, terrible,' Jean Wareham, an inhabitant of Fishpond told a BBC interviewer in November 1982. 'You feel as if you have got something pressing on your head . . . as though you are going to have something black over your eyes. You get headaches, you know, you're just so tired, so very tired.'[131] So, too, another Fishpond resident, Mrs Genge, told Roger Cook of Checkpoint: 'Since the pylons came, I've been getting quite a lot of headaches, makes you feel tired. It makes me feel quite queer at times, feeling dizzy: I certainly didn't feel like that before they came. And I want to know why. What is happening to us all?'[132]

What, indeed, is happening? Perhaps we would do well to follow Paul Brodeur's advice – namely, that if one wishes to find the root-source of a cover-up, one should follow 'the money trail'.[133] If the electricity authorities in both Britain and the United States are forced to admit that a health hazard exists, the implications could be devastating. Power lines suspended over ten thousand homes in Britain alone will have to be buried – a phenomenally expensive business – and inevitably further questions would be asked about the safety of present methods of electrical transmission for both the public and those working in industry.[134] Indeed, if the latest research is anything to go by, even burial will not be sufficient. Those living near a buried line will still be subject to enhanced magnetic fields.[135] The result could be numerous damage suits – and a bill amounting to millions of pounds.

1978 saw the publication of an American report which accused federal agencies of having been lax in setting and enforcing standards to protect the public from exposure to microwave radiation. The study, conducted by the Powerful General Office of Account (GOA), criticised the Food and Drug Administration (FDA) – the body charged with setting and monitoring safety standards for the 2 million microwave ovens in the US – for failing to regulate the microwave industry more scrupulously.[136]

In addition, the FDA was accused of not having monitored in any way the new and increasingly popular range of microwave spinoffs – from electronic burglar alarms to smoke detectors, food warmers and commercial heaters. The study recommended the Occupational Safety and Health Administration (OSHA), the Environmental Protection Agency (EPA), and the FDA join in setting a national policy on permissible exposure limits for microwave radiation.[137] Significantly, the report at least admitted that microwave radiation's 'capacity to generate heat in body levels, such as cataracts in the eyes, has been known for some time'.[138] The thermal theory was beginning to crumble; indeed, the GOA reviewed over 112 reports on microwave radiation and concluded that 'over half showed that animals and humans exposed to microwave radiation levels of 10 milliwatts per square centimetre experience biological effects, some undesirable.[139]

The GOA report is probably the first chink to appear in the microwave industry's armour – and powerful armour it has so far proved to be. Its strength lies largely in the extent to which the industry is linked to the Pentagon. Many of the Department of Defense's top officials are recruited from the microwave industry, and when administrations change, they often return to their old firms through what has become to be known as the 'revolving door'.[140] Those very firms are more often than not the Pentagon's chief suppliers of electronic equipment: thus Raytheon, the country's largest manufacturer of microwave ovens, is also the military's principal source of radar and missile guidance systems. It is, perhaps, significant that when Milton Zaret was turned down for a grant by the navy, four out of five of the 'independent' referees on the Grants Board were scientists employed by the microwave industry.[141]

In 1968, after the passage of the Radiation Control and Safety Act, the manufacturers of microwave ovens undertook to keep radiation leaks from their machines within the 10 milliwatt level, which they had voluntarily accepted as their safety standard. Yet in 1969, in a survey of microwave ovens, a third were found to be leaking above that limit: and in 1970, 10 per cent were still exceeding the standard.[142] The survey indicated that faulty door seals and safety locks were the chief cause of the problem, although poor maintenance was also to blame. The Bureau of Radiological Health was sufficiently concerned to recommend that until ovens could be tested for leaks, consumers ought to remain at arm's length from them. The microwave oven manufacturers retorted by insisting that their ovens were not leaking radiation at levels that could prove harmful. Nevertheless, the Bureau of Radiological Health decreed that as from October 1971, no oven should leak radiation at levels above 5 milliwatts per square centimetre. [143]

Milton Zaret accuses the bureau of 'regulatory duplicity' in setting that standard, maintaining that its officials met in secret with the microwave oven industry and came to a deal. [144] He points out that the bureau had known of a case where a radar worker was harmed by microwaves at far lower levels, and that the scientists who had investigated the case – one of whom was a consultant to the Bureau – had concluded that the patient had developed cataracts as a result of exposure to microwaves. [145] Strangely enough, the results of the investigation were never published and the two scientists involved were later to write that they knew of no cases of cataracts that could be definitely attributed to microwave radiation. [146]

Zaret has a powerful ally in the US Consumers Union which has always maintained that the 5 milliwatt level is still too lax. Indeed, in 1973, the union published a series of full-page newspaper advertisements, urging the public not to buy microwave ovens. The advertisement, printed on the first day of the Senate hearings on Radiation Control, stated that measurable radiation leaks had been found in fifteen leading microwave oven models; that the government's 5 milliwatt emission standard was inadequate because no research had been done on the low-level effects of microwave radiation; and that it felt the burden of proof lay with the industry to show their products were safe. [147] 'The sun is our strongest natural source of microwaves,' Zaret was to tell the hearings, echoing the words of the advertisement. 'Yet the microwave oven emission standards set by the Bureau of Radiological Health is approximately one billion times higher than the total, entire microwave spectrum given off by the sun. It is appalling that these ovens should be permitted to leak at all, let alone that the oven advertisements should encourage our children to have fun by learning to cook with them.' [148]

In Britain, the microwave oven boom has only just begun. The industry predicts confidently that sales will shoot up from their 1976 level of 10,000 units a year to 825,000 a year by 1985 – a market larger than even that for conventional cookers. [149] In the autumn of 1978, however, a programme appeared on the *World in Action* television series which dramatically altered the microwave industry's sales figures. The programme warned of the biological damage that could be done by microwaves, and almost overnight the microwave oven boom was stopped cold. The industry sent off a flurry of press releases to reassure the public, and for its part the National Radiological Protection Board made a prompt statement that microwave ovens presented no health risk. Even so, the consumer was clearly not convinced and, for a while, sales continued to plummet. [150]

However, the microwave industry has survived, and the numerous scientific warnings, though noticed briefly by the public, have not been taken up by the authorities. Indeed, under the protection of government approval, it is even now gaining back the ground it lost.

The case of the microwave oven is typical of the general problem. Where short-term interests are concerned, long-term threats are all too easily ignored. The lure of modern electronic gadgetry is a powerful one, particularly in a world where novelty is frequently confused with sophistication. For many, the advantages may indeed outweigh any suspected risks. What is certain, though, is that the dangers are much greater than is widely recognised – and it is clearly in the industry's interests to keep it that way. In the event, a change of direction might mean the demise of a billion dollar business and the tax payer having to dig deep into his pocket; that, however, may be a small price to pay to avoid the undoubted hazards of non-ionising radiation. And it is certainly a bargain compared to the costs – both financial and human – of possible genetic damage.

5

THE PESTICIDE CONSPIRACY

PESTICIDES ARE big money. Every year an estimated 2 billion tons are used throughout the world, earning some $4 billion for manufacturers in the United States alone.[1] They are sprayed on crops, on forests and on grasslands. They are used to kill insects, weeds, mites, fungi, worms and rats. Our clothes and carpets are mothproofed with them and the floorboards and paint in our houses are treated with them to prevent woodworm and fungi.[2]

But if the last thirty years have seen a boom for the pesticide industry, they have also seen an explosion of pesticide-related diseases and ecological problems. 'Some of these chemicals, such as DDT*, are now global contaminants,' reports Edward Goldsmith, editor of the *Ecologist*. 'Traces are to be found in the bodies of Antarctic penguins, in the rain, in our drinking water, and in just about all commercially produced food. Each of us has, in our body fats, traces of hundreds of different pesticides. They are in human milk, they even find their way into fertilised eggs and contaminate foetuses in their mothers' wombs.'[4] Indeed, the problem is now so acute that DDT has been found in the milk of Western mothers at levels two times higher than those recommended by the World Health Organisation (WHO) as an acceptable daily intake for adults;[5] equivalent levels of dieldrin, a close chemical cousin of DDT, were *seven* times higher than WHO

---

* The pesticide that earned considerable notoriety in the early sixties as the cause of massive environmental contamination. After a prolonged and bitter court battle, its used was banned in the USA. However, no measures have been taken by the British government to withdraw it from the market, and although its use declined in the fifties, it is now once again on the increase.[3]

recommended levels.[6] And a recent survey conducted by the US Food and Drugs Administration reports residues of the chemical in 96 per cent of all meat, fish and poultry tested; in 85 per cent of dairy products; 90 per cent of air samples: and in *all* the humans who took part in the study.[7] Dieldrin is now banned in the United States after it was found to cause cancer, but is still on sale in Great Britain.

The story of DDT, which hit the headlines in the early sixties, is widely known and scarcely needs retelling. The same is not true of the numerous other pesticides available on today's market (and there are some 45,000 brand names in the United States alone).[8] Few have been adequately tested – and many of those that have are now suspected of causing cancer, birth defects and genetic damage.[9] Not one of them has been banned in Great Britain, however, and only a handful have been withdrawn from use in the United States – usually to end up being exported to countries with less stringent environmental legislation. Scientists who report adverse health effects from the chemicals, frequently have their research suppressed and their grants cut off, whilst the safety tests on numerous pesticides have been deliberately falsified by industry-sponsored laboratories.[10] Meanwhile, the evidence that these chemicals are causing irreversible biological and environmental damage continues to mount.

Britain's most popular pesticides – known to scientists as phenoxy-herbicides – provide a particularly disquieting example. Developed during the Second World War, the phenoxy-herbicides – scientifically 2,4,5-T and 2,4-D – formed part of the allies' impressive armoury of chemical weapons. Designed as powerful pesticides, they work by promoting uncontrolled cell division. In effect, they give plants cancer.[11] Their original purpose was to destroy enemy crops and render arable land unfit for agriculture. In the event, neither chemical was used, although it is clear that – had the war gone on longer – both would have been employed by the allies.[12]

With the war over, 2,4-D and 2,4,5-T (along with other herbicides developed at the Pentagon's secret chemical warfare laboratory in Fort Detrick, Maryland), were released on to the market for more peaceful purposes and rapidly gained popularity with the public.

But the military uses of 2,4,5-T and 2,4-D were not forgotten. By 1961, with American forces fully embroiled in the Vietnam War, the

Pentagon initiated a major spraying programme – known as Operation Hades – in order to deny food to the Viet Cong guerillas and to defoliate the jungle as an insurance against ambushes. The chief spray used was a fifty-fifty mixture of 2,4,5-T and 2,4-D, code-named Agent Orange. Using giant C-123 cargo planes, the United States airforce sprayed 500,000 acres of crops and some 4.5 million acres of forest between 1962 and 1970. [13]

For its part, the Pentagon reassured the public that the herbicides being used were 'non-toxic and not dangerous to man or animals', and that 'the land is not affected for further use'. [14]

However, their reassurance proved to be unfounded. In mid-October 1969, the London *Sunday Times* carried a report on an unpublished US government study by the Bionetics Research Laboratories which incriminated 2,4,5-T as a possible cause of birth defects. Two weeks later, Dr Lee DuBridge, President Nixon's science adviser, issued a statement announcing that the government planned to curtail the military and civilian use of Agent Orange. The reason, he said, was that new studies showed a 'higher than expected number of deformities' in the offspring of mice and rats fed 2,4,5-T.' [15]

Intrigued by DuBridge's statement and the *Sunday Times* report (which had scarcely been mentioned in the US press), Thomas Whiteside, an investigative journalist for the *New Yorker,* decided to look into the use of Agent Orange a little more closely. From the outset, Whiteside, whose book on 2,4,5-T and 2,4-D, *The Withering Rain*, remains a classic, found that the scientific establishment was often disdainful of his enquiries and frequently dismissive.

'From the beginning, there was an extraordinary reluctance to discuss details of the purported ill effects of 2,4,5-T on animals,' he recalls. 'Six weeks after the publication of the DuBridge statement, a journalist who was attempting to obtain a copy of the full report made by Bionetics and to discuss its details with some of the government officials concerned, encountered hard going. At the Bionetics Laboratories, an official said that he couldn't talk about the study because "we're under wraps to the National Institutes of Health" – the government agency that had commissioned the study. Then, having been asked what the specific doses of 2,4,5-T were that were said to have increased birth defects in the foetuses of experimental animals, the Bionetics official cut off discussion by saying: "You're asking sophisticated questions that as a layman you don't have the equipment to understand the answers to.'' At the National Institutes of Health (NIH) an official who was asked for details of, or a copy of the study on 2,4,5-T replied: ''The position I'm in is that I have been requested not to distribute this information.'' He did say, however, that a continuing evaluation of the study was under way at the National Institute of Environmental Health Sciences, at Research Triangle Park, North Carolina. A telephone call to an officer in this organisation brought a response whose tone varied from wariness to downright hostility and made it clear that the officials had no intention of discussing details or results of the study with the press.'[16]

The situation was doubly sensitive because by now the civilian use of 2,4,5-T was well established. Indeed, the US Department of Health, Education and Welfare was at the time trying to assess the known health hazards of a number of pesticides (including 2,4,5-T) – and, in particular their ability to cause cancer and birth defects. To that end, the department had set up a commission – chaired by Dr Emil Mrak of the University of California and known as the Mrak Commission – on Pesticides and Their Relationship to Environmental Health.[17] Not surprisingly, when the commission's Panel on Teratogenicity (foetus deforming effects) heard about the Bionetics findings in the summer of 1969, it requested a copy of the laboratory's report. Although the National Institute of Health claim the report was made available, Dr Samuel Epstein, co-chairman of the Teratogenicity Panel, told Whiteside that the NIH refused point blank to release the full report, offering instead a statistical summary of the data. The full report, says Epstein, was only obtained 'by pulling teeth'.[18]

Indeed, Whiteside believes that, had it not been for a group of young law students, the Bionetics study might never have been made public.[19] The students were part of a team working for Ralph Nader, the consumer-protection activist, and had been assigned to investigate the role of the Food and Drugs Administration in vetting new drugs and chemicals. During the course of their investigation, one student, Anita Johnson, came across a copy of the report which had been sent to various officials at the FDA in February 1969. (Strangely, the FDA's Food Toxicology Division was not given the full report until October.)[20] Johnson summarised the report for Nader and also showed a copy to a friend at Harvard University, who, a few months later, mentioned its findings to Professor Mathew Meselson, a scientist renowned for his work on 2,4,5-T and the effects of Agent Orange. It was the first Meselson had heard of the study, but when he tried to obtain a copy, government officials told him it was 'confidential and classified' and not available to the public. Undeterred, Meselson contacted various friends in Washington and, after much effort, managed to lay his hands on a copy of the report. [21]

'What he read,' reports Whiteside, 'seemed to him to have such serious implications that he got in touch with acquaintances in the White House and also with someone in the army to alert them to the problems of 2,4,5-T in the hope that some new restrictions would be placed on its use. According to Dr Meselson, the White House people apparently didn't know until that moment that the reports on the adverse effects of 2,4,5-T even existed . . . While Dr Meselson awaited word on the matter, a colleague of his informed the press about the findings of the Bionetics report. Very shortly thereafter, Dr DuBridge made his public announcement of the proposed restrictions on the use of 2,4,5-T.' [22]

Meselson had good reason to be alarmed. The Bionetics study revealed that even extremely low doses of 2,4,5-T caused birth defects in two strains of mice and one strain of rat. Indeed, 39 per cent of laboratory rats fed 4.6 milligrams of 2,4,5-T per kilogram of body weight produced abnormal offspring. [23] At higher doses – 21.5 and 46.4 mg/kg – 80 per cent of foetuses died in the womb and a high incidence of birth defects were observed in those that survived. [24] Where 2,4,5-T was injected into mice, the results were even more alarming. 100 per cent of litters born to mothers injected with 113 mg/kg had at least one deformed offspring – and nearly 70 per cent of the mice born were defective in some respect. [25] The most common abnormalities were: lack of heads, lack of eyes, cleft palates, cystic kidneys and gastro-intestinal haemorrhages. [26]

Tests on three out of five variants (or esters) of 2,4-D revealed similar results. The five esters tested – isocytl, butyl, isopropyl, methyl and ethyl – were injected into various strains of mice at doses ranging from 46 to 150 mg/kg. Whilst the tests on the methyl ester proved inconclusive, those on butyl, isopropyl and isocytl provided firm evidence of teratogenicity. Only the ethyl ester was given a completely clean bill of health. [27]

The most significant birth defects noted in the 2,4-D tests were cleft palate, lack of eyes, incomplete bone formation in the face, lack of a lower jaw and brain tissue growing outside the cranium. [28]

The implications of these results for the use of Agent Orange were obvious. During Operation Hades the Vietnamese had been subjected to concentrations of 2,4,5-T thirteen times the level recommended as 'safe' in the United States. [29] Moreover, Whiteside has calculated that pregnant women drinking water in the areas sprayed with Agent Orange might be ingesting as much as 3 milligrams of 2,4,5-T per kilogram of body weight – 'a percentage of 2,4,5-T only slightly less than the percentage that deformed one out of every three foetuses of pregnant experimental rats' and an exposure level '600 times the concentration officially considered safe for Americans'. [30]

Indeed, by 1969 there was already considerable evidence that birth defects were occurring amongst the civilian population caught up in Operation Hades. Hospitals in the Hue district of North Vietnam, repeatedly sprayed with Agent Orange, reported that the stillbirth rate rose to 48.5 per cent and congenital malformations were found in 7.4 per cent of children. [31] There was also a significant increase in Down's syndrome, a form of mongolism. [32] Meanwhile, the Saigon Children's Hospital noted that the incidence of spina bifida increased from 1 case in 1966 to 13 in 1967; and that the number of cleft palates leapt from 2 in 1964 to 23 in 1967 – although it fell to 12 the following year. [33]

After studying the Bionetics data – subsequently confirmed by further tests at the National Institute of Environmental Health Sciences – the Mrak Commission's Panel on Teratogenicity recommended that 2,4,5-T, together with the butyl, isopropyl and isocytyl esters of 2,4-D, should 'immediately be restricted to prevent the risk of human exposure.' [34]

However, far from restricting their use, the chemical industry, when confronted with the evidence of the Bionetics study, reacted by producing new data which, on the face of it, invalidated the laboratory's results. Concentrating its defence on 2,4,5-T, the industry claimed that the birth defects observed in the Bionetics experiments were not caused by the herbicide itself, but by 2,3,7,8-tetrachlorodi-benzo-para-dioxin, an impurity found in all commercial grades of 2,4,5-T, and better known as TCDD, or simply dioxin – the chemical which wrought such terrible damage in the recent Seveso disaster.*

Even so, experiments conducted by Dow Chemicals with samples of 2,4,5-T contaminated with less than one part per million of dioxin showed a sevenfold increase in certain foetal abnormalities.[36] Dow tests on rats using 2,4-D, however, apparently revealed 'no treatment-related teratogenic responses'. Quite how Dow came to that conclusion is difficult to establish for, as Jay Lewis and John Warnock, authors of *The Other Face of 2,4,-D* point out, Dow's researchers listed a veritable catalogue of birth defects which had been observed in the rats under study – from the abnormal accumulation of fluid under the skin to water on the brain and misplaced ribs.[37]

Nonetheless, the argument that it was dioxin that was the real culprit and that 'pure' 2,4,5-T was a safe herbicide won the day: to that end, the US and British authorities set a permissible level of dioxin in commercial 2,4,5-T at 1 part in 10 million.[38] As far as the authorities were concerned, the problem was thus solved.

By raising the spectre of dioxin as their main defence against the Bionetics study, the manufacturers of 2,4,5-T and 2,4-D played a brilliant card, both because it forced their opponents to fight on terms laid down by the industry and because it effectively disarmed many of the critics' arguments. All the evidence of birth defects in Vietnam, for instance, was ruled 'out of court' because the level of dioxin in Agent Orange was 450 times higher than that found in commercial samples of 2,4,5-T.[39]

In fact, the dioxin issue is largely a red herring. Research has consistently indicated that even the purest samples of 2,4,5-T may be capable of causing birth defects, cancer and genetic damage. Experiments by the US National Institute of Environmental Health revealed a marked increase in deformities and foetal deaths – even when

---

* On 10 July 1976, an explosion wrecked a chemical plant in Seveso, northern Italy, spewing a cloud of dioxin across the surrounding area. For two weeks the authorities assured residents they were in no danger. Now they have been evacuated, and since the accident birth defects in the area have risen dramatically – from 38 per thousand in 1977 to 53 in 1978.[35] In February 1980, one of the directors of the Seveso plant was shot dead outside his home by Front Line, an off-shoot of the Red Brigade. He was accused of 'crimes against the people'.

samples of 2,4,5-T had no detectable levels of dioxin in them.[40] It is also pointed out that when 'pure' 2,4,5-T is heated, the levels of TCDD rise considerably.[41] In California, for example, foresters have frequently developed chloracne after fighting fires in areas which have been sprayed with commercial 2,4,5-T.[42] But perhaps the most significant of all, Dr Jacqueline Verret of the Food and Drugs Administration found that purified samples of 2,4,5-T and 2,4-D (which contains other dioxins than TCDD) were more teratogenic to chicken embryos than impure ones.[43]

Many environmentalists see the chemical industry's emphasis on dioxin as a means of drawing attention away from 2,4-D, by far the most widely used and profitable of the two pesticides. Earning over $2 billion in North America alone – and that figure is rising as restrictions on the use of 2,4,5-T begin to bite – the pesticide industry is understandably anxious to prevent the reputation of 2,4-D being tarnished.[44] Indeed, by honing in on the dioxin issue, the industry made it appear that 2,4-D (which contains no TCDD) had been given a clean bill of health – despite the recommendations of the Mrak Commission.

In fact, it is arguable that 2,4-D may actually be *more* hazardous than 2,4,5-T. The evidence is substantial: 2,4-D has been proved to be carcinogenic in rats;[45] cells of wheat and barley sprayed with 2,4-D have exhibited highly significant abnormalities of chromosome behaviour during cell division;[46] a 1979 study linked the spraying of the chemical to nine miscarriages in West Montana;[47] and finally tests on farm workers in British Columbia have revealed a 25-fold increase in chromosome damage after exposure to a number of herbicides, the most common of which was 2,4-D.[48]

Not surprisingly, many of those critics take the view that 2,4,5-T has been used as a scapegoat by an industry which knew that the herbicide's days were numbered. Like a mother bird shielding its young by flying away from the nest, the chemical companies are charged with cunningly drawing the environmentalists' fire away from their most profitable product by pointing the finger at 2,4,5-T. As Dr Samuel Epstein put it to me: '2,4,5-T has been made a sacrificial lamb to protect 2,4-D'.

The final nail in the coffin of 2,4,5-T was a wave of new evidence linking the chemical to a high incidence of miscarriages in Alsea, Oregon. The miscarriage rate in Alsea peaked dramatically each June, roughly three months after the area was sprayed to control forest weeds. From 1972-8, the spontaneous abortion rate was 130 per 1,000 births. In unsprayed areas it was 46 per 1,000 live births.[49] For its part, Dow Chemicals dismissed the Alsea data as 'unscientific', claiming that 'the bulk of scientific data gathered over three decades of use demonstrates that there has never been a single documented incident of human injury resulting from normal agricultural use of either 2,4,5-T or Silvex'.[50]

Residents in the Alsea area take a different view. They point to numerous incidents – dismissed by the chemical industry as 'anecdotal evidence' – in which both humans and animals have suffered health effects after spraying. Journalist Phil Keisling of the *Williamette Week*, followed up these stories and found that Alsea was not the only area in Oregon to have been affected. Peggy Hughes of nearby Allegany, for instance, has compiled a dossier which details 13 cases of cancer in the immediate area since 1971. Six of those who developed the disease lived in adjacent houses and within a quarter of a mile from a stretch of wood which had recently been sprayed and from where they drew their water. In another case, a young girl contracted a rare blood disease. A blood test showed a dramatic decrease in the girl's palates – the cells which stimulate blood-clotting – and consequently she suffered from haemorrhages. Both Silvex and 2,4-D were found in her blood.[51]

As a result of the Alsea evidence, in March 1979 (almost ten years after Dr DuBridge's announcement that use of 2,4,5-T was to be 'immediately restricted'), the Environmental Protection Agency (EPA) placed a temporary ban on the spraying of 2,4,5-T in forests, along roadsides and under power lines. The use of the chemicals on rice paddies and open ranges is still not banned, however, since the EPA claim such uses do not affect a significant number of people. In any event, it was a Pyrrhic victory for environmentalists. The use of 2,4-D remained unchecked, and by 1981, the Reagan administration was talking about 'deregulating' 2,4,5-T.[52]

In Britain the controversy has reached a stalemate. Despite the lead reluctantly taken in America by the EPA, the British Department of Agriculture has consistently denied any serious dangers attached to the use of the phenoxy-herbicides. Nonetheless, its position has been seriously undermined by a spate of press stories alleging that birth defects have been caused by 2,4,5-T and 2,4-D in Britain. One case publicised was that of Somerset farmer Geoffrey Hellier. [53]

According to Hellier, whilst making the rounds of his sheep in October 1977, he noticed a cloud drifting across his fields from a nearby Forestry Commission plantation. Approaching the plantation he saw three men clearing a path through the undergrowth. A fourth had a knapsack on his back and was dressed from head to foot in protective clothing.

Hellier claims in an affidavit that when he approached the four men, he was told to keep clear as the chemical being used was extremely dangerous. So much so, that the three men clearing the paths allegedly said that part of their job was to watch their colleague and rescue him should he collapse from the fumes of the spray. The pesticide being used, Hellier claims the workers told him, was a brush-wood killer called Silvapron-T. The active ingredient of Silvapron-T is 2,4,5-T.

For their part, the Foresty Commission workers involved deny that the spray was drifting onto Hellier's land and dispute his account of their conversation.

Aware of the controversy surrounding 2,4,5-T, Hellier became extremely concerned and immediately moved his sheep to another field, keeping a watchful eye out during the next few weeks for any sign of pesticide poisoning. At first, the sheep suffered no obvious ill effects. Then, in February 1978, just as the lambing season was about to begin, disaster struck.

'The first nineteen ewes to lamb all aborted,' recalls Hellier. 'Those ewes giving birth to twins almost invariably dropped one live and one dead lamb. The smell of those at birth indicated that they had been dead for some time.' [54]

Hellier's problems did not end there. Not long after the lambing had finished, both the ewes and their lambs began to stagger about, falling to the ground and lying there unable to get up. By late May, the majority had died. 'Altogether, I lost 29 ewes, 59 lambs and a ram in this way,' says Hellier. 'They died in very unpleasant circumstances and I was very distressed. The last ewe died in February 1979 after a prolonged illness.' [55]

Convinced that the spraying was to blame, Hellier asked his local vet to arrange a post-mortem on his ram and subsequently on a ewe. The report on the ram ended abruptly in mid-sentence. Attached to it was a note that the investigating officer at the Veterinary Investigation Service (VIS) Laboratory had apparently intended to make further comments, but that 'he was taken ill before completing the report.'[56] The VIS diagnosed the cause of the ram's staggering condition as an abscess on his rear leg. The post-mortem on the ewe noted that the animal was in a 'poor condition' and was afflicted with a number of diseases not directly related to pesticide poisoning. Although fat, brain, liver and kidney samples had been kept by the laboratory, the veterinary surgeon who carried out the post-mortem wrote that it was impossible for him to test for possible herbicide poisoning as 'there are no Ministry of Agriculture laboratories geared up to carry out tissue analysis for 2,4,5-T.'[57] He did suggest, however, that the public analyst might be able to help. Hellier has subsequently claimed that the VIS suppressed information on his case, although a Government investigation has refuted the allegation.[58]

Hellier's case would probably not have come to the public's attention had it not been for the Ecology Party. Formed in 1972, as a result of the *Ecologist* magazine's special issue, *Blueprint for Survival*, it set out to take the ideas of decentralisation, conservation of resources, negative economic growth and alternative energy sources to the hustings. By 1979, the party was strong enough to field fifty candidates at the General Election and, with membership growing at the rate of eighty new subscribing members a week, it billed itself as 'Britain's fastest growing political party'. One of those who joined ECO – as the party is popularly known – was Tony Charles, a schoolmaster from Somerset, who was quickly chosen as the party's spokesman on pesticides and other toxic chemicals. It was largely through his efforts that the well-publicised campaign to ban 2,4,5-T in Britain – now supported by the National Union of Agricultural and Allied Workers and other unions – got under way. Together with Elizabeth Sigmund, chief researcher for ECO's Standing Committee on Poisonous Chemicals and author of *Rage Against the Dying*,[59] an exposé on the use of chemical weapons, Charles has compiled an impressive dossier on the health effects of the herbicide. Among the cases he has documented are those of:[60]

■Mrs Gillian Scheltinga, who miscarried after the Forestry Commission sprayed 2,4,5-T near her home. For its part the Forestry Commission claims that Mrs Scheltinga was told which areas had been sprayed and where it was unsafe to eat blackberries. Mrs Scheltinga however told the *Guardian*[61] that she was assured that the berries were perfectly safe to eat and that although Forestry Commission workers wished to put up notices warning that spraying had taken place, the Commission refused permission. Officials also claimed that only twelve acres had been sprayed, whereas workers told Mr Scheltinga that the area was much larger.[62] The workers also directed Scheltinga to a disused mineshaft where he found eighteen used drums of 2,4,5-T and 2,4-D. Scheltinga reports that they all contained small amounts of liquid which burnt his hands. The commission, however, insists that the drums had all been sterilised before being dumped and, therefore, posed no threat to local water supplies.

■Mrs Cobbledick, the wife of a Forestry Commission sprayer, who miscarried after five months. She blames the miscarriage on her husband's use of 2,4,5-T, although the link has not been proven.[63]

■Mrs Richard Chidgey, also the wife of a Forestry Commission worker, who believes that her daughter's birth defects are due to 2,4,5-T.[64] Although the child was conceived before Mr Chidgey began working with 2,4,5-T, the Advisory Committee on Pesticides acknowledges that his wife may 'have come into contact with 2,4,5-T from her husband's working clothes between the second and eighth week of gestation'.[65]

■Barbara Young, who saw council workers spraying a playing field in Seaford, Sussex. The spray being used was 2,4-D. 'Whilst I was watching him, I felt a strange sensation in my throat,' she recalls. 'It started closing up. I was very worried about this. My throat got very sore and I couldn't swallow or speak. I felt as if I was going to die.'[66] Numerous other residents in the area complained of the same symptoms and dogs which had wandered on to the playing field began to break out in sores and develop foot eczema. A Lewis District Council official claimed that there was no cause for alarm, however, as the spray was safe and contained nothing more than an amine salt mixed with ordinary detergent. But as one correspondent pointed out in a letter to the local newspaper: 'Anyone with a smattering of chemistry knows the term "salt" covers a whole class of chemicals and "amine" is also a generic term, so the man in the street is no wiser to the real nature of the spray.'[67]

Although, in May 1980, the government did reduce the permissible levels of TCDD in commercial samples of the product from 0.1 ppm to .01 ppm, it refused to ban sales of the herbicides.[68] That decision was based on a 1979 report by the Advisory Committee on Pesticides (ACP) which argued that the risks from 2,4,5-T were negligible. 'There is no reason,' the report concludes, 'why brushkillers containing 2,4,5-T should not continue to be safely used even where the active ingredient is contaminated with TCDD to the extent of 0.1 mg/kg in the triclorophenol from which it is manufactured'.[69] In fact, 2,4,5-T remains one of the more widely used pesticides in Britain today.*

The ACP's view is not shared, however, by either the National Union of Agricultural and Allied Workers or some sixty local authorities, both of which have blacked the use of the chemical by their workforces.

Although the ACP clearly knew of the impending EPA ban when it wrote its 1979 report, it states that publication deadlines made it impossible to include a review of the Alsea data. (A subsequent report in 1980 rejects the EPA ban as unfounded.) Instead, the ACP confined itself to a review of the main criticisms against 2,4,5-T. The Vietnamese evidence is dismissed by the committee as inconclusive and the report comments that 'the short time which elapsed between the

---

* There are 14 brands of 2,4,5-T currently on sale in Britain. They are: Silvapron; Boots Bramble Brushwood and Nettle Killer; Marks Brushwood Killer; Phortox Scrub and Nettle Killer; Trioxone 50; Cambell's 2,4,5-T-MB Ester; Brushwood Emulsion; Ciba Geigy Brushwood Killer; Econal; SBK Brushwood Killer; Shell Brush Killer; Spontox; Stancide BWK75; and Synchemicals Weed and Brushkiller. All are readily available at chemists and garden centres up and down the country.

spraying of Agent Orange and the increase in liver tumours renders a causal link highly improbable'.[70] Of a study linking an abnormally high incidence of spina bifida to the spraying of 2,4,5-T in the areas of the North Island of New Zealand, the report remarks that 'investigations suggest that this effect was in two areas a chance occurrence, and that if there was a common causal factor in the third area, it was not the use of 2,4,5-T'.[71] Yet no solid evidence – apart from a reference to a New Zealand Government report – is given to support this conclusion. But perhaps the most striking omission from the report – given the ACP's contention that 2,4,5-T uncontaminated by TCDD is safe – is the total lack of any review of those studies which have shown even pure samples of the herbicide to be teratogenic. Even when, in 1982, the EEC's Scientific Committee for Pesticides recommended the banning of 2,4,5-T on woodlands and fields where the public might pick wild fruit, the British government remained adamant that the herbicide was safe. As Judith Cook and Chris Kaufman report in their book, *Portrait of a Poison*, 'the Ministry of Agriculture's immediate reaction was that such a ban would be too heavy-handed for Britain and that it would be more appropriate to close footpaths in order to keep the public away from wild foods'.

The ACP is Britain's only watchdog on pesticide use. Unlike similar agencies in America and elsewhere, however, it has no statutory powers – a situation deplored by the Royal Commission on Environmental Pollution.[72] Although pesticides are covered by the Poisons Act and the Health and Safety at Work Act, the main method of ensuring their safe use is the Pesticide Safety Precaution Scheme (PSPS), run by the ACP. Under the scheme, manufacturers of pesticides are asked to submit tests on the toxicology and health effects of any new chemicals they wish to market. If the tests are approved by the ACP and its Scientific Sub-Committee (SSC), the products are given a 'provisional' clearance, which means that they can only be used in limited areas and then only for two years. If, as a result of those field tests, no adverse effects have been noted, the ACP gives the go-ahead for a full-scale marketing of the new product.[73]

The ACP claims that the scheme is totally effective. 'Under the PSPS,' it boasts, 'manufacturers do not market pesticides in Britain unless and until the government, on the advice of the Advisory Committee, has not only 'cleared' them for safety, but also has settled what warnings should appear on the label.'[74] However, it should be noted that the PSPS is *entirely voluntary*. There is no law in Britain that prevents manufacturers (or importers) of pesticides from marketing products which have not been given the ACP seal of approval; no law which prevents farmers from using pesticides for uses for which they have not been cleared; no law which sets any standards for tests on new pesticides; and, finally, no law which requires those pesticides to be tested in the first place.[75] Although most manufacturers comply with the scheme, cases of 'banned' products being sold on a black market are not unknown.[76]

It is further open to question whether the two-year field trials for new products are totally adequate. Indeed, given the ACP's own strictures on the evidence linking Agent Orange to birth defects in Vietnam, the committee's insistence that two-year tests are sufficient seems somewhat bizarre. After all, it took six years after Agent Orange was first sprayed before birth defects showed a significant rise – a period the ACP dismissed as too short to draw any causal connections. If six years is too short a time to analyse the effects of a chemical in Vietnam, ask the critics, why should two years be adequate in Britain? Are we that different biologically from the Vietnamese? And moreover, how is it possible to pick up the cancer-causing effects of a new pesticide in two years of limited use, when most cancers take twenty to thirty years to develop?

Perhaps the most serious criticism of the PSPS is that all the data used by the ACP to judge the safety of new pesticides are provided by the very companies which have developed the products. That means that the ACP is totally reliant on tests undertaken by industries which have spent millions of pounds and years of effort bringing a chemical to the market and which stand to lose a fortune if it is banned. Moreover, those tests are not available for scrutiny by other scientists. Not even the Royal Commission on Environmental Pollution has access to the results – in one instance, the commission was refused permission to review the tests of a certain manufacturer on the grounds that 'the toxological data when quoted out of context could easily be used to mislead the public and create unnecessary alarm'.[77]

It appears also that the ACP, itself, is sometimes fed misleading information. A major reason cited by the ACP and other bodies for not banning 2,4,5-T was that only some three tons of the herbicide were being used in Great Britain each year: 2,4,5-T thus accounted for only 0.005 per cent of the total annual volume of pesticides used for crop 'protection' in Great Britain.[78] That figure went unquestioned until Dr Roger Thomas, Labour MP for Carmarthen, began to wonder why such a popular pesticide was being sold in such minute quantities. The figure just did not ring true: quite apart from anything else, he pointed out, it would mean that if the 25 herbicide brands known to contain 2,4,5-T were sharing such a tiny market, their manufacturers would be earning 'less than £4,000 a year of business for each product – not enough to pay one employee – let alone the formulation, packaging and marketing of the herbicide'. Together with two researchers, Dr Alan Williams and Gareth Wardell, both from Trinity College, Carmarthen, Dr Thomas managed to extract a detailed breakdown of imports of 2,4,5-T from the statistical office of HM Customs and Excise. They revealed that in 1979, 116 tons of the herbicide were imported into this country – some forty times more than the amount quoted by the ACP in its 2,4,5-T report. Even so, the AgroChemicals Association adamantly maintained that only 58 tons had been imported in 1979. Nonetheless, that figure was nearly twenty times the tonnage estimated by the ACP – and Dr Thomas believes the real figure may be 300 tons.[79] They point out, for example, that the Forestry Commission alone spends over £2 million a year on crop protection – enough to buy several hundred tons of 2,4,5-T, the major spray used by the commission. 'It seems clear to us,' they conclude, 'that the AgroChemicals industry in Britain has been guilty of a gross deceit of the government, of members of parliament, and of the people of this country as to the scale of use of this particular herbicide.'[80]

That episode raises a particularly disturbing question, and one that is certainly not confined to phenoxy-herbicides; if the ACP in Britain, and for that matter the EPA in America, cannot rely on industry to supply the correct statistics on its sales (a relatively simple task), can it rely on the data submitted as part of the testing procedure?

As far back as 1969, the Mrak Commission's Carcinogenicity Panel, which had just completed a review of 17 studies submitted by industry on DDT,[81] found that 14 of those studies were so badly flawed that their conclusions as to safety were, at best, invalid; at worst, misleading. To rub salt into the industry's wounds, a committee of the House of Representatives then revealed that the US Department of Agriculture had not only approved numerous pesticides for uses 'it knew . . . were practically certain to result in the illegal adulteration of food', but had also registered over 1,600 pesticides as 'safe' in spite of warnings from the Department of Health, Education and Welfare that they were dangerous to both man and the environment.[82]

For its part, the pesticide industry weathered the subsequent public storm quite comfortably, dismissing the reports as alarmist. As for the authorities, they seemed content to maintain a low profile and did little to allay the public's fears. Indeed, in 1976, an internal US government report was chiding the Environmental Protection Agency for not having improved pesticide testing procedures 'in spite of repeated warnings'.[83] The report revealed that the EPA had reviewed safety tests submitted by industry on 899 active pesticide ingredients and found that more than half of them had been so poorly tested that it was impossible to tell whether or not they were likely to be harmful to man. More alarming still, over a quarter of the pesticide ingredients reviewed – some 240 chemicals – were deemed unsafe. Indeed, 80 per cent of them were judged to be suspect carcinogens. Despite that, they were being used in almost a third of the pesticides on the market at the time.[84]

That report came a year after Dr Melvin Reuber, then a consultant pathologist to the EPA, re-examined the safety tests submitted by industry on twenty-five of the most widely used pesticides in the United States. Reuber found that, in all but one case, the data presented was, 'uniformly bad'. Worthless, it could be said, for judging the safety or otherwise of the pesticides.[85]

Reuber presented his report to the 1976 Congressional Committee Hearings on Preclinical and Clinical Testing in the Pharmaceutical Industry. Testifying at the same hearings was John Quarles, deputy administrator of the EPA, whose evidence amply backed up Reuber's findings. The committee, chaired by Senator Edward Kennedy, had already heard disturbing reports (see Chapter 7) that countless safety tests conducted on toxic chemicals and drugs had been falsified in order to get them approved for sale. Quarles confirmed that the same problem was widespread amongst laboratories testing pesticide products. Indeed, he not only acknowledged that studies showing the dangers of certain pesticides had been withheld from the EPA, but also warned that some laboratories 'might be so dependent on a pesticide producer for contract work that [their] independent judgement could be impaired by the close economic relationship' – and that 'in certain cases a laboratory might intentionally misrepresent test results at the request of the manufacturer'. [86]

We have already seen how this affected the phenoxy-herbicide issue. There are several other cases of similar magnitude. In 1975, for instance, the EPA had received information that the Chicago-based Velsicol Chemical Corporation had wilfully concealed the results of laboratory tests which showed that chlordane and heptachlor, two insecticides manufactured by the company, caused liver cancer in rats. That information resulted in six Velsicol executives being charged, in 1977, with conspiracy to 'defraud the United States and conceal material facts from the US Environmental Protection Agency'. The indictment alleged that Velsicol's management had been told of the pesticides' dangers by its own consultants, but had chosen to suppress the findings for three years. [87]

Whether the allegations were true will never be known, for the company's lawyers had the case dismissed on procedural grounds. [88] What is certain, however, is that it was largely as a result of tests submitted by Velsicol purporting to show the two insecticides were safe, that the Mrak Commission's recommendation that they be restricted (based on an earlier report by the US Federal Drugs Administration) was ignored. The Velsicol tests, carried out by the Kettering Laboratories of the University of Cincinnati and the International Research and Development Corporation (IRDC) of Michigan, revealed that both heptachlor and chlordane caused 'nodules' in the livers of laboratory rats, but it was denied that these were cancerous. Subsequently, an independent re-examination of the livers preserved at IRDC by five pathologists (headed by Dr Melvin Reuber, then a professor at the University of Maryland) concluded that those 'nodules' were, in fact, malignant tumours and that the incidence of liver cancer amongst the test rats was abnormally high. [89]

Moreover, an investigation by the Environmental Protection Agency discovered that during a separate 1966 study, which Velsicol also claimed gave heptachlor a clean bill of health, the Kettering Laboratories had removed 'an unknown number of subcutaneous tumours from the test animals' without either diagnosing or reporting them.[90]

The EPA announced its decision to ban all uses of heptachlor and chlordane in November 1974. Inevitably, Velsicol contested the decision and after a long court battle the ruling was reversed. The EPA appealed and finally won the case, but the victory was qualified; under concerted pressure from the pesticide industry they were forced to concede a 'phased withdrawal' of both pesticides from the market, the production of 7.25 million pounds of both heptachlor and chlordane being permitted every year until September 1982.[91]

The cases of 2,4,5-T, heptachlor and chlordane are by no means exceptional. Similar examples of duplicity by the pesticide industry abound:

■The dangers of dibromochloropropane (DBCP) – used against roundworm and mites – were first reported in 1958.[92] Yet it was not until 1977, after workers manufacturing the pesticide were found to be sterile and to have reduced sperm counts, that those dangers were publicly acknowledged.[93] The 1958 study showed that DBCP caused severe shrivelling of the testicles in laboratory rats. Shell Chemicals were informed of the findings in a confidential report from researchers at the University of California's School of Medicine in 1958. A study by Dow Chemicals yielded similar results. Yet, even after these reports were published in 1961, neither company saw fit to issue a public warning about the dangers of their products.[94]

Confronted with this evidence in 1977, an executive of Occidental Chemicals admitted that he had known about the Dow study, but claimed that the company had been unaware of its significance.

'I've just talked to two scientists who are familiar with the work,' he told an investigator, 'and they both say: "Heck, we just didn't draw the conclusion that there'd be sterility from the fact that the testicles were shrivelling up!"'[95]

Much of the research on DBCP has been carried out at the

University of California. 'The professor who directed the research, Dr Charles Hine, has throughout his tenure at the university been a paid consultant to Shell,' reports Ralph Lightstone, a lawyer for the California Rural Legal Assistance Programme, who testified that before a 1980 Congressional committee, chaired by John Miller, on the DBCP cover-up. 'By his own admission, during those DBCP research years, Shell directed his research priorities. Meanwhile, Shell has been making annual 'gifts' to the university for toxicological research. The gifts request that Hine oversees the research.'[96]

Shell, who funded the research on DBCP through a series of twenty-seven grants to the university, made no bones about the results they expected. 'We are interested,' wrote W.E. McCauley, an executive for the company, 'in the development of data to support the use of Nemagon Soil Fumigant (DBCP).'[97]

■In early 1975, a doctor in Hopewell, Virginia, sent a blood sample for analysis at the Centre for Disease Control (CDC) in Atlanta, Georgia. The sample came from a Mr D. Gilbert, a patient who worked at Life Science Products, a local factory manufacturing the insecticide Kepone under contract to Allied Chemicals.[98] The CDC found that Gilbert's blood was contaminated with high levels of kepone (32 parts per million) and immediately informed the Virginia State epidemiologist. 72 of the 150 workers at the plant were found to be similarly contaminated, with 30 of them requiring immediate hospital treatment.[99] Like Gilbert, they showed the classic symptoms of kepone poisoning; weight loss, involuntary twitching of the eyeballs and tremors – symptoms known locally as the 'kepone shakes'.

The plant was immediately closed down. Subsequent investigations not only revealed that the surrounding area was thoroughly polluted with kepone, but also that Life Science had discharged the chemical through the local sewer system – with the city council's knowledge – and contaminated both the James River and Chesapeake Bay (see Chapter 2).[100] Moreover, it emerged that Allied Chemicals had first learned of the toxic effects of kepone as far back as 1962.[101] Tests conducted by the Medical College of Virginia, under contract to the company, had shown unequivocal evidence that the chemical accumulated in animal tissue; that it caused liver damage, possible damage to the reproductive system and certain harm to the central nervous system; and, finally, that it was carcinogenic – a finding reinforced by the National Cancer Institute.[102, 103] A year after the Hopewell plant closed, Allied was fined $13.2 million for continuing to sell kepone whilst knowing its toxicity and for breaking federal water pollution standards.[104]

■A 1967 study, carried out by Shell Chemical's Tunstall Laboratories in Great Britain and kept from the public for six years, showed that both the pesticide dieldrin and its close chemical cousin, aldrin, were carcinogenic.[105]

The two insecticides, widely used on corn crops despite evidence that the insects they were designed to kill had developed genetic resistance to them, were finally banned in the US in 1975 after four years of court hearings.[106] At those hearings, Shell argued that studies – dating as far back as 1962 – which showed the chemicals to cause cancer in mice, should be disregarded as it did not consider the mouse to be a suitable animal for cancer tests.[107] Despite this, the company had been quite happy to cite negative studies using mice as evidence that dieldrin and aldrin were safe. An independent review of those studies, however, revealed that numerous tumours which had been described as 'benign' were, in fact, malignant.[108]

In a final effort to avoid a ban on the two insecticides, Shell produced a study of workers exposed to 'high levels' of aldrin and dieldrin which, it was claimed, showed no evidence of excess cancers. The study, undertaken at a Shell insecticide factory in Pernis, Holland, was re-examined by a panel of leading epidemiologists. 'It was unanimously agreed that the study was so flawed and inadequate that it was not possible to draw any conclusions at all from it,' reports Dr Samuel Epstein. 'Not only was it based on too few workers, exposed and observed for too short a period for any significant excess of cancer other than a catastrophic one to be noted, but it was also clear from blood analyses that over 30 per cent of the workers had never had any substantial exposure to aldrin and dieldrin in the workplace.'[109]

In the event, Shell lost its battle. In September 1974, Judge Herbert Perlman announced that, in his opinion, the continued use of dieldrin and aldrin constituted an unreasonable risk to the American public. 'There is no fooling around,' he told the court. 'The major issue is cancer.'[110] Despite that hazard, however, the EPA allowed the company to sell off its existing stocks – the agency simply could not afford to indemnify Shell against loss of sales.[111]

For its part, the British Advisory Commission on Pesticides rejected outright Perlman's decision and the subsequent EPA ban. Indeed, both chemicals continue to be sold in Britain – as in most other countries – despite increasing evidence of their harm to both humans and the general environment.

Robert Van den Bosch was a distinguished entomologist, who devoted most of his career to the development of 'integrated pest management', a system of pest control which relies on natural rather than chemical controls to keep insect populations in check. He was also an outspoken critic of what he termed 'the pesticide mafia' – that powerful group of vested interests which keep modern agriculture 'hooked' on the use of pesticides despite the mounting evidence of their hazards. As he puts it in his book, *The Pesticide Conspiracy*, published shortly before his death in 1979: 'The pro-pesticide mafia operates much in the manner of those in its Italian namesake. It has its *famiglie*, its *capi*, its *consiglieri*, its *soldati*, its *avocati*, its lobbyists, its front organisations, its PR apparatus, and its "hit men". It owns politicians, bureaucrats, researchers, administrators, and elements in the media, and it can break those who don't conform. In other words, it is a virtual duplicate of the other *mafia* that pervade and dominate so much of contemporary American society.'[112]

This mafia's most powerful weapon is money and it uses it ruthlessly. By manipulating the system of grants to those universities carrying out research on pest-control, the pesticide industry ensures that many researchers are effectively in its pocket, afraid of stepping out of line for fear of losing their funding. Those mavericks who refuse to tailor their research results to the dictates of the industry often find themselves harassed, even intimidated and, certainly, threatened. A case in point is that of a young researcher at the University of California who found that commercial samples of canned tomatoes which had been heavily sprayed contained as many insects as samples which had received no pesticides. 'To prove his point,' reports Van den Bosch, 'he set up an experiment in which he deliberately infested tomatoes with insects, processed and canned them, and then compared the level of insect contamination in his bugged tomatoes with that in canned juice available in the supermarket. He found no difference . . . Next, he set out to publish the results of his study. But the tomato canners got wind of this and sent a delegation to the university administration to complain about the manuscript and to threaten withdrawal of grants were the paper to be published. The university brass, upset by this prospect, suggested to the entomologist that he back off. His description of his reaction to this subtle administrative arm-twisting reflects the widespread reality of life in the agricultural experiment station: 'Hell, Van, what could I do? I was just a little guy raising a family and up for promotion. You better believe I tore that manuscript up'' '[113]

Despite the evidence that the pesticide industry has frequently attempted to intimidate scientists, manipulate data and suppress unsympathetic research results, many claim that the benefits of pesticides are so enormous that we should not gripe at a few isolated cases of duplicity on the part of a generally honest industry. But are such claims justified? Would mankind really be worse off without pesticides?

There is a tragic irony to our escalating use of pesticides. Far from alleviating the problem of pests, pesticides have actually resulted in a dramatic increase in the number of pest outbreaks. Indeed, according to the EPA, the amount of crops destroyed by pests before harvesting has doubled since the 1930s – despite a twelvefold increase in the tonnage of pesticides used by farmers.[114] The reasons for this are clear. To begin with, insects have an astounding ability to develop genetic resistance to the pesticides with which they are sprayed. Often turning over a new generation every week, insects exhibit incredible 'genetic plasticity' which enables them to adapt rapidly to changing environmental circumstances.[115] No spraying programme can completely eradicate an entire population of pests in one fell swoop.

Inevitably, some pests will survive and among the survivors will be those whose genetic make-up was such that they were unaffected by the spray. They may, for instance, have been able to manufacture a particular enzyme which detoxified the pesticide; or, again, some quirk in their behaviour may have protected them from the poison. Provided that the number of survivors is sufficient to allow breeding to continue, the extraordinary adaptiveness of the evolutionary process will ensure that a higher proportion of the next generation is afforded the same genetic protection – and the species will rapidly develop resistance to the particular pesticide being used. Indeed, it is now estimated that some 364 species of pests are now resistant to nine of the major pesticides available to farmers.[116]

That problem is compounded by the very destructive nature of pesticides. 'Modern insecticides are *biocides*,' comments Robert Van den Bosch. 'That is, by design, they kill a wide spectrum of animals. This is the root cause of the insecticide treadmill on which so many farmers now find themselves, for the chemicals kill good bugs as well as bad ones. Thus, if not intelligently employed, they can trigger a bug backlash by interfering with the balance of nature which occurs even in our most severe crop monocultures. For example, when applied to a crop, a biocide kills not only pests but also other species in the insect community, including the natural enemies that restrain noxious species. Often, the natural enemies suffer excessively, first because they are generally less robust than the pest species and, second, because the insecticides deplete their food supply (i.e. the pest species) so that they starve or leave the fields. As a result, insecticide spraying frequently creates a virtual biotic vacuum in which the surviving or reinvading pests, free of significant natural enemy attack, explode. Such post-spraying explosions are often double-barrelled, in that they not only involve the resurgence of target pests, but also the eruption of previously minor species, which had been fully suppressed by natural enemies. The frequent outcome is a raging multiple pest outbreak, more damaging than that for which the original pest-control measure was undertaken. Predictably, the grower or other insecticide user, in order to salvage his cotton, fir trees, rosebuds or whatever, reapplies insecticides and when this triggers still another multipest outbreak, he sprays again. This is the genesis of the insecticide treadmill . . .'[117]

It is also the beginning of the end for our environment: indeed, the scale of ecological havoc being wrought by pesticides is already alarming.

That depradation was first highlighted by Rachel Carson in her book *Silent Spring.*[118] Now recognised as a classic, *Silent Spring* provoked a vitriolic response from the pesticide industry when first published in 1961. Indeed, attempts were made to dissuade Houghton Mifflin from publishing it. Those who questioned the use of pesticides (and by inference, Rachel Carson) were accused of being unwitting pawns for 'sinister influences' out to wreck Western agriculture and reduce the free-world's food production to 'east-curtain parity'. The company behind those insinuations was Velsicol Chemicals.[119]

Many pesticides – particularly DDT and other chlorinated hydro-carbons – are insoluble in water, with the result that they tend to accumulate in the fatty tissues of those plants and animals which eat them. Clearly, the larger the animal the more pesticide it can store and consequently, as one moved up the 'food chain', the concentration in fatty tissues increases – a process known to scientists as 'biomagnifi-cation'. The process is best illustrated by the wholesale contamination of the aquatic food chain in California's Clear Lake after it was sprayed with DDD, a close chemical cousin of DDT, in order to control gnats. Levels of the chemical in the water were as low as 0.02 parts per million; plankton and other microscopic organisms feeding in the lake, however, accumulated DDD residues at 4 parts per million; fish eating the plankton concentrated the pesticide still further – to levels as high as 2,000 parts per million; and birds feeding on the fish were found to be contaminated with 80,000 times the level of DDD present in the lake with the result that thousands died.[120] Because pesticides such as DDD and DDT are highly persistent, only breaking down into their constituent chemicals after long periods, this biomagnification can continue for years after spraying has ceased. Nor do ecosystems have to have been sprayed directly for such contamination to take place. Persistent pesticides, like DDT, can be released into the atmosphere through evaporation and then deposited back on the land in droplets of rain – often miles from where they were originally used.[121] Indeed, one study has shown that Swedish soils contain some 3,300 tons of DDT, more than twice the entire quantity of DDT used in Sweden over the past twenty years.[122] Even soils which had never been treated contained traces of the chemical at an average of 0.1 parts per million – five times the level present in the waters of Clear Lake, California.

But perhaps the greatest threat of biomagnification lies in its effects on the foods we eat. Almost all the foods on sale in Great Britain now contains pesticide residues. 'In the last available survey,' reports Edward Goldsmith, 'levels of different pesticides in different food-stuffs that were regarded as being of any significance (classified as "reporting levels") were noted. Only one foodstuff – fourteen samples of honey – was free of residues of organo-chlorine pesticides. A large percentage of foods had levels that contained residues above reporting level – 41 per cent of samples of hard cheese for instance, 28 per cent of soft cheese, 45 per cent of butter, 33 per cent of infant food, 65 per cent of strawberries. The average daily intake of organo-chlorine pesticides from the consumption of 1,700 grammes of food was 0.056 milligrams.'[123] Goldsmith also notes with alarm that the World Health Organisation is now resigned to mothers' milk and baby foods being contaminated with the pesticides aldrin and dieldrin. Indeed, WHO's expert committee on contaminants in food concluded that it is now 'impossible to produce milk or baby foods entirely free from aldrin and dieldrin'. [124]

Even when a pesticide is banned, however, the consumer is not protected from eating food contaminated by it. All too often, industry (ever adept at exploiting a setback) simply exports the outlawed pesticide elsewhere – usually to the Third World. As David Weir and Mark Shapiro of the San Francisco based Institute for Food and Development Policy point out in their book, *Circle of Poison*: 'Massive advertising campaigns by the multinational pesticide corporations – Dow, Shell, Chevron – have turned the Third World into not only a booming growth market for pesticides but also a dumping ground. Dozens of pesticides too dangerous for unrestricted use in the United States are shipped to underdeveloped countries.'[125] Indeed, according to a 1979 report by the US General Accounting Office, 'at least 25 per cent of pesticide exports (from the United States) are products that are banned, heavily restricted or never registered for use'. [127] Those pesticides include kepone, DDT, heptachlor, aldrin, dieldrin, chlordane and DBCP. In some cases the cynicism displayed by companies is galling: 'There's no problem with the ban of DBCP within the United States,' an executive of Amvac, an

American chemical supplier, told Weir and Shapiro. 'In fact, it was the best thing that could have happened to us. You can't sell it here anymore but you can still sell it anywhere else. Our big market has always been exports anyway.' [127]

One consequence of such exports is that much of the food imported into America from the Third World is contaminated with pesticide residues. Thus milk from Guatemala was found by the General Accounting Office to be contaminated with DDT at levels 90 times in excess of US safety limits; in 1976 the US Department of Agriculture refused entry to some 500,000 pounds of DDT-contaminated beef from El Salvador after it was found to contain residues of the pesticide which were 19 times higher than those permitted under US law. [128]

Yet, as Weir and Shapiro report, such seizures are rare: 'Despite the widespread contamination of imported food, inspectors (from the Food and Drugs Administration) rarely seize shipments or refuse them entry. Instead a small sample is removed for analysis while the rest of the shipment proceeds to the marketplace – and the consumer. The rationale is that perishable food would spoil if held until the tests were known. But by the time the test results are available – showing dieldrin or parathion or DDT residues – the food has already found its way to our stomachs. Recalls are difficult . . . During one 15-month period, government investigators found that half of all imported food identified by the FDA as pesticide-contaminated was marketed without any penalties to the importers or warnings to consumers . . . Peppers from a shipment that was sent on to supermarkets turned out to have 29 times more pesticide residues than allowed by US law.' [129]

Just five days before he left office, President Jimmy Carter signed an 'executive order' which would have introduced legislation to curb the trade in banned pesticides. On February 17th 1982, President Reagan revoked the order. [130]

In itself, Reagan's action is a sign of the cynicism of governments throughout the Western world. For there is no question that the trade in banned pesticides is responsible for thousands of deaths and poisonings in the Third World. According to the World Health Organisation (WHO), 500,000 people are poisoned in the Third World every year by pesticides and 5,000 of those die – that is, one poisoning a minute and one death every hour and 45 minutes. [131] Moreover, those figures are probably underestimated.

Thus, although more than 1,300 pesticide-related poisonings (all sufficiently severe to warrant medical treatment) were reported in California in 1975, Dr Ephraim Kahn, chief of the Epidemiological Studies Laboratory of the California Department of Public Health, estimates that those reported cases probably represent only one per cent of the total number of poisonings.[132] If the number of poisonings can be so underestimated in the USA, then it is likely that the figures for pesticide poisonings in the Third World – where many people do not even have access to a doctor, let alone a statistician – are even wider off the mark.

All in all, then, our food and our environment is thoroughly contaminated with thousands of different pesticides. Nobody knows the biological effects of that cocktail of chemicals. Nobody knows the ultimate fate of persistent chemicals in their environment or their effects on the structure and health of the soil. What is certain, however, is that the price for our futile war against the insect will be paid not in the dollars and pounds so dearly loved by the chemical industry, but in increased rates of cancer birth defects, genetic abnormalities and environmental degradation. Is it a price we are really prepared to pay?

6
ACID RAIN:
THE POISON FROM THE SKIES

SCIENTISTS SEE it as one of many 'atmospheric depositions'. To the media, it is 'a silent scourge'. But, for the man in the street, it has become known as 'acid rain'. At times more acid than vinegar, it has corroded buildings, killed fish, rotted women's tights and turned the hair of elderly matrons a fashionable punk-rock green. Already it has transformed lakes into lifeless bodies of deceptively clear water: it has stunted and debilitated the growth of trees; and it is destroying crops throughout the industrial world. Indeed, it is not for nothing that acid rain has been described as 'one of the most devastating forms of pollution imaginable, an insidious malaria of the biosphere'.[1] Others have gone so far as to suggest that if action is not taken soon, acid rain could bring about 'an ecological holocaust'.[2]

The cause of the destruction is air pollution in the form of sulphur dioxide and nitrogen oxide. Released as gases into the atmosphere through the burning of coal and oil, the minute particles of sulphur dioxide and nitrogen oxide react with water and sunlight to form droplets of sulphuric and nitric acid. Once in the troposphere, those acids can be transported by prevailing winds for distances of up to 1000 kilometres in a few days before being rained down upon the earth.

Pollution from one country can thus damage crops, forests and lakes in another country many hundreds of miles away. Indeed, it is estimated that West Germany, for example, receives 90,000 tons of sulphur dioxide from England, 50,000 tons from France, 40,000 tons from Belgium, 30,000 tons from Holland and 90,000 tons from other unknown sources.[3] Meanwhile, West Germany itself pours its own pollution into the atmosphere, contaminating other countries. Small wonder, then, that the eminent Swedish scientist, Svante Oden, has accused the nations of Europe of waging 'chemical warfare' against each other.

In itself, acid rain is nothing new. As early as 1662, the English social historian, J. Evelyn, noted that industrial pollution was damaging plants. Moreover, he suggested, much of that pollution was coming across the Channel from France. The solution to the problem, he said, was to build taller chimney stacks so that the pollution would be spread to 'more distant parts'.[4] A century later, a certain Mr Hales wrote a treatise in which he described the air around industrial centres as being 'full of acid and sulphurous particles'. But the first full description of acid rain and its effects came in 1852 when an English chemist, Robert Angus Smith, took samples of rain around Manchester and analysed its chemical content. Smith saw clearly that the rain samples he took from near the city centre were quite different from those he took from the surrounding countryside. He conluded: 'We may therefore find three kinds of air – that with carbonate of ammonia in the fields at a distance, that with sulphate of ammonia in the suburbs, and that with sulphuric acid or acid sulphate in town.'[5] Twenty years later, in his book *Air and Rain: the Beginnings of a Chemical Climatology*, Smith coined the term 'acid rain'.[6]

Smith's book was a remarkable piece of scholarship: indeed, according to Ellis Cowling, Chairman of the US National Atmospheric Deposition Programme, it 'enunciated many of the principal ideas that are part of our present understanding (of the problem)'. In particular, 'Smith demonstrated that precipitation chemistry is influenced by such factors as coal combustion, decomposition or organic matter, wind trajectories, proximity to the sea, and the amount and frequency of rain or snow. Smith proposed detailed procedures for the proper collection and chemical analysis of precipitation. He also noted damage by acid rain to plants and materials and commented on the atmospheric deposition of arsenic, copper and other metals in industrial regions. Unfortunately, however, Smith's pioneering and prophetic book apparently has been overlooked by essentially every subsequent investigator.'[7]

Perhaps that is not surprising – for no-one (least of all industry) likes to be told that their activities are threatening disaster. Time and time again, the warnings of eminent scientists have gone unheeded. Indeed even today it is claimed that we do not know enough about acid rain to take action to prevent it: thus, Anna Gorsuch, the Administrator of the US Environmental Protection Agency told a symposium on acid rain in October 1982: 'Our experience of recent years should teach us not to rush in with quick fixes where we know we have an inadequate understanding of existing conditions.'[8]

Such statements are no doubt music to the ears of industry. Yet, as one Canadian official complained recently, 'we cannot wait for a perfect understanding of the acid rain phenomenon before moving to control it . . . how many more lakes have to die before we get the message?'[9]

How many indeed? For whilst governments procrastinate, the environmental toll of acid rain continues to mount.

■As lakes become increasingly acid, so their waters become incapable of supporting life. 'When the acidity of waters begins to rise,' explains ecologist Erik Eckholm, 'fish reproduction is impaired and calcium in fish skeletons becomes depleted causing malformed "humpback" fish. Acidic waters also unlock aluminium from surrounding soils, which then builds up on fish gills. As water pH falls below 5.5*, smaller species of crustaceans, plankton, molluscs and flies begin to disappear. At a pH of 5.0 the decomposition of organic matter, the foundation of the aquatic food chain, is undermined. Below a pH of 4.5 all fish are dead and the only remaining life is a mat of algae, moss and fungus. Lacking organic matter, the water of an acidified lake assumes the crystal clarity of a swimming pool – a deceptive beauty indeed.'[10]

Some 10,000 lakes in Sweden now have a pH value below 6.0 and 5,000 lakes have a pH value of 5.0.[11] In the Adirondacks – a remote mountainous region of the Eastern United States – 90 per cent of the lakes above 2,000 feet are now so acid that few fish can survive in them. Fifty years ago, fewer than 4 per cent of the lakes in the region were acidic.[12] Ten per cent of New England's lakes are now so acid that it is no longer considered worthwhile restocking them with fish. According to *Time* magazine: 'Canadian environmental officials project the loss of 48,000 lakes by the end of the

---

* pH is a measure of acidity. A pH of 7.0 is neutral: the lower the pH, the higher the acidity.

century if nothing is done to curb acid rain. Already they estimate that 2,000 to 4,000 lakes in Ontario have become so acidified that they can no longer support trout and bass, and some 1,300 more in Quebec are in the process of being destroyed.'[13] Even before the lakes actually die, the fish in them can be rendered unfit for human consumption. For accompanying acid rain are other pollutants – including such heavy metals as lead, cadmium, zinc and mercury. Moreover, where soils contain these heavy metals, acid rain leaches them out, releasing them into nearby waterways.[14] Inevitably, they are then taken up by fish and – in the case of mercury – converted into methyl mercury. In that organic form, mercury is highly toxic. Indeed, by 1982, fishing had been banned in 100 Swedish lakes because the mercury levels in fish were too high.[15]

■Two thirds of the total land area of North America now receives acid rain.[16] At times the rain over New England – where the acid rain pollution is so bad that the area has been described as the 'garbage can of the US' – is 30 to 40 times more acid than 'normal' rain – and levels of acidity 500 times that of unpolluted rain have been recorded.[17] Nor has Britain escaped the menace. As Fred Pearce reports in *New Scientist*: 'In the Lake District in Cumbria, scientists at the North West Water Authority attributed at least one large haul of dead fish in the River Esk to acid rain. But such chance finds may be just the tip of the effects in Britain . . . At Loch Fashally in the Scottish Grampian region, the average pH of rain fell from 5.2 in 1962 to 4.2 in the mid-1970s. That represents a 10-fold increase in acidity . . . Scotland has the dubious distinction of measuring the most acid rain ever measured. At Pitlocherie, a Ministry of Agriculture, Fisheries and Food station has measured the rain from one particularly virulent thunderstorm to have a pH of 2.4 – more acid than vinegar.'[18]

■In West Germany, acid rain is killing trees in the Black Forest and elsewhere. 'Across Bavaria, some 1,500 hectares of forests have died in the past five years,' reported Fred Pearce in 1982. 'Another 80,000 hectares of forests in Bavaria and Baden-Wurttemberg are seriously damaged. Some German forests have taken from industry doses of sulphur amounting to 100 kilograms or more per hectare every year for more than a century.'[19] Ironically, in its first stages, acid rain 'poisoning' actually induces trees to grow more rapidly – for they benefit from the rain's high nitrogen content. That stage, however, is followed by what is known as 'die-back'. The forest soils rapidly lose their ability to neutralise the acid in the rain. The acid then begins to accumulate and, as it builds up, so it leaches out vital minerals and nutrients. 'The loss of (those) nutrients', explains Fred Pearce, 'slows the growth of trees and damages the wood, but much worse soon follows. As the nutrients are removed so the sulphate begins to combine with metals in the soil. The most important is aluminium, which is present in huge quantities in most soils. Normally, aluminium is harmlessly bound with organic materials. But when these links are severed and the metal goes into solution with sulphate it becomes very toxic . . . Acute poisoning occurs as the aluminium starts to inhibit the division of cells in the roots of the trees and destroy its defences against disease organisms . . . The toxins invade, damaging the cells as they go. The tree cannot seal the damaged root system and the spores of the bacteria, fungi, viruses and other pathogens invade and work their way in. In this way secondary diseases begin. The tree is doomed. Death will come slowly by a mixture of starvation, disease and poisoning.'[20]

■In the USA alone, an estimated 1 billion dollars worth of crops are destroyed each year through acid rain. The worst affected are grains like alfalfa and certain root and leaf crops.[21] No-one knows for certain exactly the effect of acid rain on soil organisms – but if the history of its effects on forests is anything to go by, it is likely to be extremely deleterious.

Whilst the forests and lakes die and crops are destroyed, a propaganda war has broken out between those countries which are being polluted and those which are doing the polluting. Indeed the issue of acid rain is now a source of bitter wrangling between such countries as Canada, the United States, Sweden and Great Britain. For their part, the polluters wish for more time to research the problem before taking action; the polluted, however, have demanded immediate steps to curb emissions of sulphur dioxide and nitrogen oxide. Such anti-pollution measures would cost industry dear – £1,500 to remove one ton of sulphur, adding up to a total bill of £1.5 billion for Britain's Trent Valley power stations alone – and, perhaps inevitably, there has been much lobbying by industry to stop any new regulations being introduced.

That lobbying reached a pitch in the summer of 1982 at a conference in Stockholm held to discuss means of tackling the problem of acid rain. But if anyone was expecting a co-ordinated 'clean-up' programme to emerge from the conference, they were to be sorely disappointed. Stonewalling and a cynical exploitation of scientific uncertainties were the order of the day – at least as far as the polluting countries (notably Britain and the US) were concerned. Thus Britain's Central Electricity Generating Board – whose coal- and oil-fired stations have been blamed for much of the sulphur dioxide 'exported' by Britain via the North Sea to Scandinavia – flatly denied either that the link between acid rain and the acidification of lakes had been proved or that sulphur dioxide emissions in Britain were contaminating Europe. Thus, the Board insisted that, 'only if it can be proved that pollutants transported over long distances play an important part in the decline of fish stocks in Scandinavia will it be necessary to consider reduction of pollution at source'. [22]

That ostrich-like attitude – flying as it does in the face of ten years of research to the contrary – found few supporters at Stockholm. Indeed, according to Fred Pearce, not even the British government (which in the past has taken much the same line as the CEGB) felt able to support the Board's position. [23] But whilst British officials now acknowledge that British sulphur is damaging European lakes and soils, they have baulked at taking action. Thus, when it was suggested by the Swedish and Canadian governments, that European and North American power companies should cut sulphur emissions by 50 per cent, the reply was predictable: to implement such a cut would not only be uneconomic but also, quite possibly, ineffective. As Giles Shaw, then Under-Secretary of State at the Department of the Environment, put it to the conference: 'How can we justify the additional costs of fitting equipment to remove sulphur from the emissions of existing power stations? We cannot be sure that they will be effective in curing the environmental problems . . . A large reduction in emissions in one country may have only a marginal effect on another country.' [24] Echoing that view, Kathleen Bennett of the US Environmental Protection Agency, argued that it would be 'scientifically insupportable' to push for stricter sulphur controls because 'the scientific community cannot tell us yet where and when to reduce emissions and by how much'.[25]

Both Bennett and Shaw have a point: scientists do not know the exact relationship between a given cut in sulphur emissions and a given fall in the acidity of rain. Some believe that the relationship is a direct one – that a 50 per cent reduction in sulphur emissions will bring a 50 per cent fall in acidity – whilst others argue that the problem is more complex. But whilst it is certainly right to point out the scientific uncertainties, it is surely unforgivable to exploit them quite as unscrupulously as the British and US governments have done. For uncertainty is hardly an excuse for inaction. Who, after all, would suggest leaving someone tied to a railway line simply because no-one knew the exact time the next train would pass?

Moreover, whilst the British government remains adamant that further research is needed on acid rain, it has done precious little to fund such research. Indeed, in April 1982, the government *cut off* research grants (worth some £120,000) to the Institute of Terrestrial Ecology; the grants were to have been used to study the effects of sulphur dioxide on forest flora.[26] In the event, those funds were reinstated following the release of a report by Warren Springs Laboratory which showed that acid rain is not only falling in Britain itself but that in some areas the acidity is 'of the same order as in the high input areas of Scandinavia and North America.'[27] It is also thought that pressure was exerted to reinstate the grants by government scientists who had become increasingly concerned at the evidence presented at the Stockholm conference on the effects of acid rain on forests.[28] Nonetheless, later in the year, the British government refused to fund research into the effects of acid rain on crops – as a result of which the Institute of Terrestrial Ecology lost a further grant. It would thus appear that whilst government scientists (who are supposed to advise the government) are growing increasingly alarmed over acid rain, the government itself would prefer not to hear their advice. Politics, rather than science, are winning the day. Indeed, of the £4 million earmarked each year for acid rain research half goes to CEGB, the very industry under scrutiny.

Meanwhile, in the United States, there is considerable evidence that President Reagan – who had already gone back on President Carter's commitment to cut sulphur emissions – is attempting to stack the research cards in industry's favour. Thus, the Reagan Administration declared itself unsatisfied with a group set up by the National Academy of Sciences to review the literature on acid rain as part of a joint research programme with Canada. One reason for the Administration's dissatisfaction is that the National Academy of Sciences had previously published a report arguing that sulphur dioxide emissions should be reduced by 50 per cent. 'Because some authors of that report now serve on the NAS joint committee with Canada,' reports Eliot Marshall in *Science*, 'the Reagan Administration apparently did not think the latter would give favourable advice. The White House went shopping for other experts. James McAvoy, former White House adviser on this issue, told the *New York Times* that he thought the NAS group might not give an ''objective'' review. One non-government expert at the centre of this controversy says, ''the Administration simply wanted more control over the results.'' '[29]

Industry is undoubtedly delighted. Meanwhile vast tracts of Canada are devastated, whilst in Britain the government procrastinates even as the acid falls. But can we really afford to give industry the benefit of the doubt whilst we wait to marshall all the facts and figures on acid rain? Can we really let economics rule over common sense? Or should we follow West Germany's example and cut sulphur emissions by 50 per cent because 'action not taken today will cost us a lot more in a few years time'. Above all, can we afford to go on using the atmosphere as a rubbish dump? Undoubtedly the fate of large areas of both Europe and North America depends on the answer to that question. But if the government and the CEGB's record is anything to go by, it is doubtful that the British public will receive an honest answer.

7

THALIDOMIDE AND AFTER

EACH AND every one of us has taken a drug at some time in our lives. It may have been as innocuous as aspirin – it could have been a stronger, prescribed drug such as Valium or Mogadon. Either way, it had a chemical base and as such was potentially harmful. By and large, we assume that our major pharmaceutical companies are honest enough to test those drugs to the most stringent standards before they are released on to the market. But the truth is rather different. The evidence suggests that, so long as research costs have to be recuperated from the profits of drug companies, pharmaceutical products which are known to be dangerous are being sold. The result has often been catastrophic.

In the early sixties, an epidemic of birth defects swept the world. Its cause was a wonder drug known as thalidomide. Developed by Chemie Grunenthal, a German pharmaceutical company, thalidomide had been aggressively marketed in forty-six countries as a safe, non-toxic sedative with no side effects. Taken between the fifth and eighth week of pregnancy, however, its effects were far from calming. One pill was sufficient to cause the most disturbing deformities in the growing foetus. Babies were born with flipper-like arms and legs, brain damage and appalling injuries to the intestinal tract. Others were blind, deaf, autistic or epileptic. Today, some 8,000 children have grown up in the shadow of thalidomide's fallout – and many others have died from its poisonous legacy.

For its part, Grunenthal argues that the thalidomide disaster was the result of a lack of scientific knowledge for which it could not be possibly held responsible. At the time, it was claimed, no one knew that drugs could cross the placental barrier and harm a foetus without harming the mother; all the appropriate tests had been performed, and it was impossible to have predicted the drug's terrifying side effects from them. Those myths have now been exploded, thanks largely to the diligent detective work of the *Sunday Times*' Insight team. In its book on the thalidomide affair, *Suffer the Children*, [1] the Insight team published internal documents from Grunenthal which reveal that the company – together with its associates who marketed the drug under licence – knew about the adverse effects of thalidomide for some time before it was withdrawn from the market. Those documents provide powerful evidence that Grunenthal acted in a manner which can at best be described as naïve, at worst dishonest.

The first real evidence that thalidomide was not the wonder drug that Grunenthal claimed it to be came during clinical trials in the mid-fifties. Three out of nine doctors to whom the drug was sent for tests reported adverse effects amongst patients ranging from constipation to a 'hangover' feeling. One senior practitioner warned that 'in his patients, thalidomide produced giddiness, nausea, wakefulness instead of sleepiness, and addiction after about three weeks'. [2] Nonetheless, Grunenthal produced a report which gave thalidomide a clean bill of health. What they omitted to say, however, was that the most favourable reports for the drug came from scientists who were retained by the company. Moreover, despite experimental evidence that thalidomide interfered with the working of the thyroid gland – an effect known at the time to be associated with birth defects – Grunenthal failed to carry out teratogenic tests. Contrary to the company's claims, such tests were by no means extraordinary in the fifties.* Further, there is no question that scientists did in fact know

---

* Comments the Insight team: 'Grunenthal, in order to sell its drug, thought it useful to give the impression that a clinical trial with pregnant women had been made. That certainly strengthened the "hypothesis of safety" as publicly perceived. Had Grunenthal actually thought to have such a trial conducted, and had it been competently organised, it would have been very likely that teratogenic effects could have been picked up with suffering confined to a dozen cases or so. But Grunenthal not only failed to conduct a clinical trial to examine thalidomide's safety in pregnancy, it failed as well to carry out any reproductive studies on animals. Other drug companies *at that time* . . . were doing such studies . . . '

Elsewhere, Insight points out: 'It was in no way unusual for reproductive studies

that substances with thalidomide's molecular weight could cross the placental barrier and Grunenthal's failure to perform reproductive studies appears both extraordinary and unforgivable.

By the late fifties, reports that thalidomide caused peripheral neuritis – a severe affliction of the nervous system which causes numbness of the joints, cramp and lack of co-ordination – were beginning to flood into Grunenthal's head office. One doctor who was particularly concerned about this effect was Ralf Voss, a nerve specialist from Dusseldorf. But when he wrote to the company asking whether thalidomide could affect the peripheral nervous system, he was assured: 'Happily, we can tell you that such disadvantages have not been brought to our notice.'[4] In fact, two months earlier, Pharmakolor AG of Basle, Switzerland had reported: 'To date, twenty well-known doctors have told our representatives that when they themselves, or their patients, took one tablet of thalidomide they found themselves still under its effects the next morning, suffering from considerable sickness, involuntary trembling of the hands, etc. Dr Ludwig, head of the second medical department, Burgershospital, Basle, told us yesterday that he gave his wife a tablet [of thalidomide]. He adds: "Once and never again. This is a terrible drug." '[5]

At the time, thalidomide could be bought across the counter but, by early 1960, the pressure was on Grunenthal to place the sale of the drug on prescription. As the Insight team reports, it was not a prospect that appealed to the company:

'Unfortunately we are now receiving strong letters on the side effects of thalidomide, as well as letters from doctors and pharmacists who want to put it on prescription,' the company's sales department wrote. "From our side, everything must be done to avoid this, since the substantial amount of our volume comes from over-the-counter sales."

'Grunenthal's sales manager, Dr Klaus Winandi, suggested the

---

to be made with drugs in the days before thalidomide was invented, though practice varied among companies and, of course, among different drugs. There would be no point in doing reproductive studies with a drug designed to combat the effects of senility. But the scientific record makes it clear that many scientists considered that drugs in the sedative/hypnotic/tranquiliser bracket . . . should be checked for reproductive dangers.'[3]

tactics: the company should appeal to doctors and pharmacists' profit motivation. Representatives should spell out to them how much they stood to lose: "Bring economic aspects into conversation, and this will provide an opportunity for explaining to the doctor that such a harmless sleeping draught should really remain exempt from prescription . . . In a similar way, one will probably also be able to meet any objections from pharmacists. A hint can be dropped that the consumption of thalidomide will boost sales, which would certainly drop if compulsory prescription were to be introduced."

'While the company's salesmen set about this task, the clinical research department was also doing its best to protect the drug that Grunenthal came to call "this apple of our eye". Dr Gunther Michael, head of the section, warned: "Sooner or later we will not be able to stop publication of the side effects of Contergan [the trade name under which thalidomide was being sold]. We are therefore anxious to get as many positive pieces of work as possible." To this end, some rather remote stones were not left unturned. On 30 March 1960, a Grunenthal representative reported that initial approaches to a doctor in Iran had been unsuccessful. "However, since the Iranian doctor is very materialistic in his outlook, concrete results should be forthcoming soon." The head office was left to interpret this cryptic sentence in any way it wished. In point of fact, the representative in Iran seemed to be pursuing the right course because what Grunenthal wanted above all was *quick* results. The company spelled out its policy on trials in a letter to the Portuguese licensee, Firma Paracelsia, of Oporto: "To be quite clear about it: a quick publication, perhaps in three months, with the reports of fifteen to twenty successful cases who have tolerated the drug well, is more important to us than a broadly based, large work that will not appear for eight to twelve months. From this, you can see what kind of testers we have in mind."

'. . . Pending favourable reports, Grunenthal did what it could to suppress or delay publication of unfavourable ones. Its tactics with Dr Frenkel, [a] neurologist from Konigstein, were not atypical. When it learned that he was preparing a paper for publication describing his experiences with twenty patients, all of whom, he believed, had thalidomide-induced peripheral neuritis, two representatives paid him a visit. It would be a great help to the company, they said, if he were to withhold his article. Dr Frenkel said he had already sent it to *Medizinishe Welt*. Then withdraw it, the Grunenthal men suggested. Frenkel refused. Would he at least delay it? No, Frenkel said.

'But the publication of the report was delayed, seemingly inexplicably: it was some time before the reason emerged. A Grunenthal memorandum explained: "The friendly connection with Dr Matis [editor of *Medizinishe Welt*] contributed to the delay in treatment of the submitted manuscript." [Dr Matis later denied that he had allowed Grunenthal to influence him, but agreed that he had forwarded Frenkel's paper to Grunenthal for its comments. Many scientists have experienced that when an editor submits their papers to hostile reviewers, there is often a delay in publication.] In the meantime Matis published in *Medizinishe Welt* an article written by a woman doctor who had previously done some work for Grunenthal. It noted: "The particular advantages of Contergan reside in its atoxity and in the lack of side effects after long use." '[6]

That cover-up would continue throughout the early sixties. In 1961, for instance, Dr Voss, the neurologist who first questioned the drug's affects on the nervous system, gave a speech at a medical meeting in Dusseldorf warning of the dangers of thalidomide. A Grunenthal representative, Johann Goeden, responded by suggesting that the drug be mixed with other sedatives so that 'if it proves impossible to keep things in the dark or to ward off attacks, any alleged side effects could then be attributed to the other preparations. But heaven help us if this expedient turns into a boomerang.'[7] Later, according to Insight, Goeden reported to Grunenthal that he 'had visited a clinic in Cologne where . . . [he] . . . took the opportunity to explain our standpoint over the peripheral neuritis problem . . . and did [his] best to foster confusion on this subject'.[8]

More was to come. As reports of peripheral neuritis continued to flood in, so Grunenthal's stance stiffened:

'Doctors who questioned Grunenthal's attitude,' reports Insight, 'were abused as troublemakers. Dr Hubert Gigglberger of Regensburg, who told Grunenthal that it was "irresponsible" not to have withdrawn the drug, and that he doubted the company's trust-worthiness, was labelled "troublemaker No. 1" of the South German area. The local company representative wrote to [Grunenthal]: "We have to pull out this sick tooth before the infection spreads". Could the service of a private detective help?

'Two months earlier, Grunenthal had hired such a man, Ernst Jahnke of Essen, to place under surveillance certain patients with peripheral neuritis who might raise compensation claims against the company. The aim was to try to prevent any civil lawsuits because of the damage that the cases, with their attendant publicity, could cause Grunenthal. Now the company ordered the detective to extend his attentions to doctors who criticised thalidomide . . . '[9]

Meanwhile, in Britain, Distillers (Biochemical Company) Limited (DCBL) – a subsidiary of the company which manufactures Gordon's Gin and Johnny Walker whisky – had bought the licence for thalidomide and was marketing it under the trade name Distival. Relying on Grunenthal's testing, Distillers had done little independent research on the drug themselves, yet saw its reputed 'non-toxity' as a particularly powerful selling point. One man who was concerned about the drug, however, was George Somers, Distillers' pharmacologist, and a man whom even the company's severest critics exonerate for his part in the thalidomide affair. Early in 1959, Somers found that a liquid preparation of the drug was, in fact, poisonous – a finding that constituted a direct attack on Distillers's claim that the drug was non-toxic. Moreover, Somers also had evidence that thalidomide could cause adverse effects in patients, and duly informed the company. Insight describes the reaction:

'Throughout June 1960 a series of memos flew among DCBL executives. Surprisingly, they seem mainly concerned not, as one might imagine, with giving serious consideration to withdrawing the drug pending further tests, but rather with anticipating publication in medical journals of the fact that Distival was toxic.

'C.N. Brown [the deputy of Dr Walter Kennedy, chief medical adviser to Distillers] thought the time had come when it would be "wise" to modify DCBL's claims for Distival. He suggested substituting for "no demonstrable toxicity" the phrase "low or very low toxic effects''. It was decided that all references such as ''non-toxic'' and ''free from toxicity'' would be deleted from DCBL publications about Distival – but not until the next reprinting!

'Somers was the only DCBL man out of step and he was pressing for publication of all findings: ''I think you are of the opinion that a danger exists and we should present the facts as soon as possible.'' But DCBL was unhappy about losing its major claim for Distival – that it was a safe sedative or hypnotic. At least one executive, the managing director, D.J. Hayman, made it clear he thought the safety angle was getting out of proportion. And as late as May 1961, more than a year after Somers had discovered that [a liquid preparation of thalidomide] was toxic, Hayman admitted that DCBL was still circulating from time to time an abstract of Somers' earlier report, which said that he had been unable to find that thalidomide had any lethal dose whatsoever.

'Somers appears to have done his best to persuade DCBL to publish all his latest findings. He tried the ''self-interest'' approach: ''Some day someone is going to make the observations we have made with different formulations of thalidomide. They may publish them and cause us some damage. If we have already drawn attention to these matters . . . we will be in a much stronger position.''

'Hayman was unmoved: ''I cannot see any reason why we should extend the debate outside the scope of Grunenthal-DCBL.''

' . . . DCBL was now heavily occupied with a sudden flush of reports of more cases of peripheral neuritis. January and February 1961 saw more and more doctors concerned with this severe and frequently incurable side effect of thalidomide. February, alone, brought 8 definite and 5 suspected cases to the London office of DCBL in Wimbledon, and the company began to consider at last putting ''a little more emphasis'' on the risk of peripheral neuritis ''in the hope that the number of cases will diminish if doctors are aware of the possibility''.

'This plan did not meet with the unqualified approval of the sales side of the company. J. Paton, a sales executive, wrote: ''It is not our job to educate the medical profession how to look out for various conditions. From a sales promotion point of view the more we write on this side effect, the more it is likely to get out of perspective.'' It is not hard to speculate about the reasons for this alarming attitude. By the end of March 1961, DCBL had sold nearly 64 million thalidomide tablets. April turned out to be the best month for sales in three years.' [10]

The behaviour of Richardson-Merrell, the American company which bought the franchise for thalidomide, was little better than that of either Grunenthal or Distillers. By the grace of God, however, the drug was never marketed in the United States and the tragedy that overtook Europe and many other countries was averted. The credit for keeping thalidomide off the market goes entirely to Frances Kelsey, a pharmacologist at the Food and Drugs Administration in Washington. Her husband, who also worked for the FDA, had reviewed the drug tests submitted on thalidomide by the company. He concluded: 'The section entitled "Chemical Comparisons of Thalidomide and Glutethimide" is an interesting collection of meaningless, pseudo-scientific jargon, apparently intended to impress chemically unsophisticated readers.' Kelsey went on to describe the company's absorption tests as 'completely meaningless'. [11]

More than the inadequacy of the tests that Richardson-Merrell had submitted, Frances Kelsey was concerned that the company had failed to report evidence that thalidomide caused peripheral neuritis – a side effect which was gaining wide publicity in the British medical press. No doubt she would have been even more concerned to know, as we have seen, that although Richardson-Merrell's pharmacologists knew that thalidomide could theoretically cross the placental barrier, they had performed no reproductive tests to see whether in fact it did. [12]

In any event, Frances Kelsey turned down Richardson-Merrell's application to market the drug.

However, despite Kelsey's stand, the United States did not entirely escape the thalidomide tragedy. Before submitting its application to market the drug to the FDA, Richardson-Merrell had conducted a massive clinical study in which some 20,000 people were exposed to thalidomide. As a result, between ten and sixteen children were born with birth defects. That figure is necessarily imprecise as no one knows for certain how many women were actually given the drug. In fact, as the Insight team points out, the clinical trial was conducted with scant regard for accepted medical procedures:

'Actually, the trials were not clinical ones in the true sense of the term. To begin with, the "investigational program" – as it was called within the company – was run by the sales and marketing division, not the medical department, and although the medical department had a veto over the salesmen's choice of doctors to carry out the trials, the very fact that the salesmen were allowed to select the doctors was unusual in the American drug industry. Also, the salesmen were told not to offer placebos – fake pills that are a vital part of a blind trial needed to ensure that the patient's reaction is genuine and not imagined – but to wait until the doctor requested them himself. In fact, Richardson-Merrell's approach must have seemed casual to many of the doctors, for when thalidomide was eventually withdrawn, it emerged that several hundred of them could not get in touch with patients to whom they had given the drug because they had kept no records of the fact. In short, several of the main reasons for the investigational program seem to have been not clinical at all, but to develop a marketable product, to perfect the best possible sales story for the national introduction of thalidomide into the United States, to encourage favourable publication of thalidomide's properties, and to establish throughout the country local studies whose results could be spread among hospital staff members.' [13]

But the cover-up was not confined to clinical tests. Even when the effects of thalidomide became evident, the manufacturers refused to acknowledge their responsibility.

The link between thalidomide and the horrifying crop of birth defects sweeping those countries where the drug was on sale was first established by Dr William McBride, an obstetrician from Sydney, Australia. McBride had come to suspect the drug was teratogenic after three of his patients gave birth to deformed children. All three had taken Distival – the trade name for thalidomide which was being marketed in Australia by a subsidiary of Distillers – during their pregnancy. McBride confided his fears to Dr John Newlinds, the medical supervisor at Sydney's Women's Hospital, the largest obstetrics hospital in Australia. Newlinds, himself, had been increasingly concerned at the spate of deformed babies being delivered in the hospital – by then running at a rate three times the national average – and when McBride urged him to withdraw the drug from the hospital's pharmacy, he readily agreed. McBride then telephoned Distillers and told them that, in his opinion, they should stop promoting thalidomide until more was known about its possible teratogenic effects. Distillers took note of his remarks and promised to relay his fears to their head office in London. Inexplicably, London was not informed for another five months. [14]

Meanwhile, in Germany, Professor Widukind Lenz, head of the Children's Clinic at Hamburg University, had reached the same conclusion as McBride: there was no doubt in his mind that thalidomide was a powerful teratogen. On 16 October 1961, he wrote to Grunenthal:

'Since about 1957 a certain type of deformity has occurred in West Germany with increasing frequency. It is a matter, in the first place, of serious defects in the limbs, especially the arms, which are usually mere stumps with two to four fingers or none at all. These malformations are in part combined with serious leg defects and also with the absence of the outer ear, closure of the auditory passages, heart trouble and blocking of the oesophagus. There have always been deformities of this kind, but their incidence has certainly been less than 1 in 50,000, probably less than 1 in 100,000. During 1959, 1960 and 1961, the increase in the number of deformities of the type described has been so marked that it has been noticed in numerous places . . . Last year 1 or 2 out of every 1,000 infants born in Hamburg were deformed in this way. A very intensive search in Hamburg for any factor that could possibly be associated with the occurrence of these deformities has led to the discovery of one single factor regularly present in all these cases. In each of the 14 cases of which I have a reliable account, thalidomide had been taken during the early months of pregnancy . . . In view of the incalculable human, psychological, legal and financial consequences of this problem, it is, in my opinion, indefensible to wait for a strict scientific proof of the harmfulness or harmlessness, as the case may be, of [thalidomide]. I consider it necessary to withdraw the medicament from sale immediately until its harmlessness as a teratogenic agent in man is conclusively proved.' [15]

Ten days later, Grunenthal received a report of McBride's findings, belatedly forwarded to them by London. Even though several company officials now urged that the drug be withdrawn from sale, Dr Heinrich Mueckter, who led the team which first synthesised thalidomide, remained intransigent. The next day, however, *Welt am Sonntag* published a front-page story reporting Lenz's fears. The article finally forced Grunenthal to take thalidomide off the market.

Not that the company gave up easily. 'Grunenthal was determined not to lose its wonder drug without a struggle,' reports Insight. 'It argued that even if thalidomide did cross the placenta, there was still no evidence that it was responsible for deformed births. Anyone who agreed with this proposition was encouraged to say so publicly. Those who disagreed were described within Grunenthal as "trouble-makers, opportunists or fanatics". The company's real virulence was reserved for Lenz, and a campaign was started to discredit him and to "influence the press for our purpose".' [16]

By now, however, the evidence against thalidomide was overwhelming. Most damning of all was a test carried out by Dr Somers of Distillers on white rabbits. Of 18 babies born after four rabbits had been fed thalidomide during early pregnancy, 13 were hideously deformed. [17] When Grunenthal heard of these results, it urged Somers not to publish his findings – a suggestion which Somers ignored despite pressure from some of his colleagues at Distillers. Indeed, after Somers' report appeared in the *Lancet,* one senior executive made it quite plain that he expected company scientists 'to steer a very careful course between the advancement of scientific knowledge through scientific publications and the bad publicity that these are likely to generate through the popular press and elsewhere'. [18]

In fact, Distillers did not stop selling thalidomide altogether until December 1962, although it did withdraw it from sale to pregnant women. Some other countries, however, delayed taking even that step. 'Governments and social institutions not only failed to keep the drug off the market, but in some cases did not act quickly even when its effects were realised,' reports Insight. 'Official indolence in Japan meant that several hundred thalidomide babies were born long after the world learned of the danger; for more than a year after thalidomide had been with withdrawn from sale or prescription in other countries, the Japanese authorities allowed mothers in Japan to go on taking it without prescription. In Sweden, the drug was withdrawn but the authorities did not warn mothers against using thalidomide pills already released – at least five babies were born needlessly crippled – and the drug was kept on sale in Argentina by the Swedish manufacturer for three months after it had been withdrawn in Sweden. Thalidomide stayed on the market in Canada for three months after it had been withdrawn in Britain and Germany, but this sorry record was surpassed in Italy. Thalidomide was sold under ten different trade names there and some pills were still on sale ten months after the withdrawal of the drug in Germany.'[19]

Nor did the sorry tale of thalidomide end with the drug's withdrawal from the market. The parents of thalidomide children still faced protracted court cases to gain compensation for their children's injuries. In Britain, that court battle lasted twelve acrimonious years, during which Distillers placed enormous pressure on the parents to accept an offer which turned out to be a twentieth of what they were finally awarded. The *Sunday Times* was intimately involved in that court case after it was prevented from publishing the full story behind the thalidomide tragedy – from Grunenthal's 'testing' of the drug to the attempts to suppress information on its adverse side-effects by Britain's antiquated laws on contempt of court. It need hardly be said, however, that the £28 million awarded to Britain's thalidomide victims scarcely recompenses the psychological and physical stress suffered by that generation of babies whose only sin was that they were in their mother's womb when a thoroughly toxic drug happened to be on the market. Far more comforting would be the relief of knowing that such a disaster could never happen again. Unfortunately, it appears that indifference on the part of drug companies was not a prerogative of the fifties. It would seem to be the hallmark of the industry.

Senator Kennedy: Dr 31 worked on drugs for three different pharmaceutical companies: Roche, Knoll and Endo. The data submitted to Knoll turned out to be an exact duplicate of the data submitted to Endo the preceding year with only the dates changed. The data submitted in these studies was entirely fabricated: is that correct?
Dr Hensley: That is correct.

Senator Kennedy: Would you review what Dr 31 told the Food and Drug Administration (FDA) inspectors happened to him that caused him to lose his data?

Dr Hensley: Dr 31 characterised himself as a compulsive worker. He stated that he really had done the studies but he just had so much to do that he felt that he had to take the work with him on a picnic and had the data in the rowboat with him. And the rowboat allegedly capsized. The data went to the bottom in a metal box and was not retrievable. He did admit to us during the inspection that he had falsified the data. He had tried to make it as close to the original as he could, he said, but it was false.

Senator Kennedy: Did this doctor not ask two nurses to corroborate the fact that they were with him when the boat capsized?

Dr Hensley: Yes, he did.

Senator Kennedy: Were the nurses, in fact, with him?

Dr Hensley: No. Mrs J. said one day during the fall of 1977, Dr 31 came to her work area and said he wanted to talk with her. She said her desk was in a public area rather than a private office, and Dr 31 indicated that he wanted to talk with her alone. She said they went into the vacant doctor's office and the doctor closed the door. She said the doctor told her that an investigator from the Food and Drug Administration would see her the next day, and the doctor wanted her to confirm the statement he had made to the investigator that the two families were in a boating accident at a local lake and some of the doctor's research papers were destroyed. Mrs J said the doctor appeared to be very frightened. Mrs J said she told the doctor she had never been on the boat with the family and she could not confirm his statement to the FDA investigator, whereupon he became very angry.

I could read a similar statement from another nurse, but it is the same type of thing.

Senator Kennedy: Where did Dr 31 claim to have gone to medical school?

Dr Hensley: The University of Saigon, during the Japanese occupation.

Senator Kennedy: What did the FDA learn when it tried to find out if, in fact, the doctor had gone to the University of Saigon or to the Paris campus of the University of Saigon?

Dr Hensley: We had quite a bit of help from the Veterans Administration. We were able to locate two or three witnesses, one a fellow who happened to have a list of graduates at the University of Saigon for the appropriate years, and two others who were doctors who graduated in the same class as this physician allegedly graduated. It would appear that the doctor never went to the University of Saigon.

Senator Kennedy: Is there any evidence that Dr 31 is in fact a doctor?

Dr Hensley: Not at all. There is, in fact, a communication from the doctor to the French affiliate of the university: 'If anybody asks, please say I went there.' [20]

That cross-examination took place when Dr Hensley of the FDA's Scientific Investigation Service testified before Congressional hearings into Preclinical and Clinical Testing by the Pharmaceutical Industry, chaired by Senator Edward Kennedy. Dr 31 was supposed to have been testing the reaction of patients to a new psychoactive drug. Such tests are frequently carried out by doctors and the results of their research are critical to any decision to market a drug. If Dr 31's case was an isolated incident, we might have little to worry about. However, the evidence presented to the Kennedy Committee suggests that such dishonesty is widespread and extends beyond doctors monitoring the side effects of drugs for the pharmaceutical industry. Numerous laboratories testing the safety of the thousand or so new chemicals we release into the environment each year, are now seen to have manipulated their research results to give harmful products a clean bill of health.

As early as 1966, Dr James Goddard, then commissioner of the FDA, warned that the quality of industry-sponsored new chemicals was often 'dismal'; that in many cases unfavourable data was being deliberately withheld from the FDA; and that companies seeking scientists to research new products frequently chose those 'who were known to be more concerned about industry friendships than developing good data.' [21] Nor is the falsification of research results a purely American phenomenon. A 1976 survey by Dr Ian St James Roberts, a lecturer at the University of London, showed that British scientists are just as prone to dishonesty as their American colleagues. 'The most frequent kind of cheating,' reports Roberts, 'is data massage where findings are eased and stretched to fit the desired results.'[22]

Neither the British nor the American authorities have yet come to grips with the problem, claiming that with 16,000 scientists in the US alone, it is almost impossible to police all laboratories. Others take a more sceptical view. Senator Gaylord Nelson of Tennessee, for instance, has no illusions as to the real cause of the delay in introducing legislation to tighten controls in industry-sponsored research. 'Industry is big and it is powerful,' he told a 1976 Senate committee (also chaired by Edward Kennedy) which investigated the problem. 'You have got the chemical industry which is powerful. You have got the drug companies and they are powerful. You have got the people who make food additives and they are powerful.'[23]

Indeed they are; and the evidence is that they are frequently unscrupulous. All too often research which shows a new product in a bad light is suppressed, falsified or ignored; companies take calculated decisions to market drugs and chemicals they know to be unsafe; and scientists who speak out to warn the public of these dangers are intimidated. Consider a few recent examples:

■Schering AG is the Berlin based company which first launched the oral contraceptive pill in Europe. It is also the largest manufacturer of Primados, a hormone pregnancy test which has been used by millions of women. In Britain, the drug is produced by a subsidiary company, Schering Chemicals Ltd of Burgess Hill, Sussex.

In 1967, Dr Isabel Gall, a researcher at Queen Mary's Hospital at Carshalton in Surrey, published a study linking the incidence of spina bifida – a crippling spine disease – in babies to the use of hormone pregnancy tests by their mothers. The report was read by the research director at Schering Chemicals, Dr Michael Briggs, who became extremely concerned – not least because the most widely used brands of the contraceptive pill contain, in varying strengths, the same hormones contained in Primados and other similar pregnancy tests. If Dr Gall's analysis was correct, millions of women were even then at risk.

Briggs immediately arranged for his own epidemiological survey. He contacted a mathematician at the University of Sussex, Dennis

Cooke, and asked him to match the figures for sales of Primados in Britain to a detailed breakdown of birth defects throughout the country. On 2 November 1967, Cooke reported that he had found 'a strong correlation' between the incidence of birth defects and the sales of the drug. Briggs at once informed executives at Schering Chemicals and his superiors in Berlin.

. 'Throughout what followed, Schering's German head office took a consistent line: it attacked uncomfortable news and tried to protect Primados,' comments Oliver Gillie, the *Sunday Times* journalist who first broke the story. 'Berlin's first line of defence against Briggs' news was to respond that in Germany, sales of the drug did not correlate with birth abnormalities. But when Briggs sent the German figures to Cooke, the mathematician pointed out that, unlike those in Britain, German statistics do not record *all* birth defects, only deaths from abnormalities. Berlin's calculations were misleading.'[24] So, too, was the head office's second line of defence: studies were in progress, it was claimed, to test the effects of Primados on the litters of mice and rabbits. In fact, the studies were not on Primados, but on Schering's range of contraceptive pills.

By this time, the directors of Schering Chemicals – who behaved impeccably throughout the affair, stopping promotion of the drug once they heard of Briggs' study – were becoming extremely alarmed at Berlin's attitude. On 6 June 1968, the company's medical directors, Dr Alan Pitchford and Dr Patrick Eye, wrote to their counterpart in Germany: 'We must reach a decision regarding . . . Primados and its possible relationship to foetal abnormalities,' they urged. 'As manufacturers, it is our moral duty to do all possible to ensure the safety of the preparations which we market. Where suspicion of any kind has been aroused by an investigator whose ability and integrity cannot lightly be challenged, the onus of proof must lie with us. It is for us to establish that the drug is safe to use . . . '[25]

Clearly unimpressed by that argument, Schering's head office remained intransigent. No action would be taken over the drug. Rebuffed yet again, Pitchford then turned to the British Committee on the Safety of Drugs (CSD), the official watchdog of the pharmaceutical industry in the United Kingdom, in an attempt to get the drug withdrawn. The committee refused to act, however, claiming that there was 'insufficient information' to justify a ban. Just what was meant by that phrase is unclear, for the evidence against Primados was mounting almost daily.

'In January 1969,' reports Gillie, 'a survey by the Royal College of General Practitioners revealed an apparent increase in abortions among women taking the hormone drugs. The college circulated the survey privately among drug companies and, remarkably, even though the author of the survey, Dr Norman Dean, was sufficiently alarmed by his results to recommend withdrawal of the drug, the current president of the college, Dr Ekkehard von Kuenssberg, felt able to write to Schering; "I hope you won't feel worried" by what he called Dean's "personal opinion . . . " ' [26]

Even when the CSD was replaced by the Committee on Safety of Medicines (CSM), no action was taken – despite a study by two committee members which showed that women using hormone pregnancy tests gave birth to a higher percentage of deformed babies. Indeed, it was not until Oliver Gillie first revealed the dangers of Primados that the CSM finally agreed to warn doctors that the drug might cause birth defects. 'Schering at once responded by attaching a red warning label to the Primados packets available in Britain,' reports Gillie. 'Even that was clearly inadequate. According to independent market research figures, sales of Primados and other hormone pregnancy test drugs in Britain fell by a third in Britain following these warnings. Yet some 40,000 women were still prescribed the drugs as a pregnancy test in 1975, and some 25,000 had it in 1976. Even in 1977 – after a second safety warning from the Committee – 6,000 women in Britain took the drug as a pregnancy test . . . and Schering acknowledge that they did not attach red warning labels to Primados sold outside Britain.' [27]

■On 24 January 1980, FDA Commissioner, Dr Jere Goyen, received a letter urging him to ask the US Justice Department to press criminal charges against Smith, Kline and French (SKF), a major drug company in the United States. The letter, written by Dr Sydney Wolfe of the Nader Health Research Group, alleged that SKF had failed to report 12 cases of liver damage caused by the anti-hypertensive drug, Selacryn, within the statutory fifteen-day period.[28] Although the cases were included in a seven-volume quarterly report submitted by the company to the FDA in November 1979, they were not picked up by the agency until January 1980. When the FDA discovered them, it immediately took the drug off the market, whereupon SKF announced evidence of 40 other cases, including 5 deaths.[29]

Although the company discovered the dangers of the drug in July 1979 – in one case it was 105 days before it reported an incidence of liver damage – it nonetheless embarked on a massive promotion campaign in September, sending free samples of the drug to every doctor in the United States. Its advertising slogan was: 'First step drug for treating hypertension: Prescribe with confidence' and sales leapt from 3,000 bottles in May 1979, to 80,000 in October. During that period, some 300,000 patients are estimated to have taken the drug; according to FDA sources, about 1 in 500 of them will damage their liver and 60 per cent will have suffered from jaundice. An independent expert on drug-induced liver damage estimates that 1 in every 10 of those who developed both liver damage and jaundice will probably die.[30]

■Benurestat is an enzyme inhibitor developed by the US-based Norwich Pharmical Company for dissolving kidney stones. The drug was tested on volunteer patients at McAlister Prison, Oklahoma, in 1973. Even before the results of a low-dose study had been analysed, a high-dose study was begun. In the event, that study had to be discontinued because half the volunteers succumbed to diarrhoea, abdominal pains and liver poisoning.

James Downey, a prisoner at McAlister, volunteered for the tests because it 'was just about the only way of getting money'. In 1975, he testified before a Congressional committee that he had been told that the drug had been tested on animals but had produced no adverse effects other than 'something that went wrong' with bone marrow functions. In fact, studies had also revealed that Benurestat caused liver damage in dogs.[31]

Downey was also told that there would be a doctor on call at all times during the experiment. When he fell ill on a Friday night, however, he discovered that all the doctors had gone away for the weekend. He was left in the care of a researcher from the prison's

Medical Research Unit. 'He told me I had measles,' Downey recalls. 'I was dehydrated and real bad and he sent me back to work.' In fact, Downey had acute hepatitis. [32]

■Triflocin, developed by Lederle Laboratories, is a drug which promotes urine excretion. In August 1968, the company was given the go-ahead to test the drug on humans, even though long-term animal studies had not been completed. Those studies eventually revealed that Triflocin caused bladder tumours in rats – but the results were not revealed to the FDA for nine months. Several years later, the case was re-examined by the US Bureau of Drugs which recommended that the company be prosecuted. The recommendation was turned down, however, on the grounds that too long a period had elapsed since the offence was committed. [33]

■The wife of a doctor testified before the 1979 Kennedy hearings on clinical drug trials that, on several occasions, she had helped her husband falsify reports on his patients' reactions to new drugs. In one study, her husband was supplied with two bottles of pills; one containing the drug to be tested; the other, a placebo, a pill with no active medical properties. Against the express orders of the drug company for which he was undertaking the study, the doctor found out which bottle contained which pill. With that knowledge, he was then able to fill out fictitious medical reports – filling in results which would be in the normal range of reactions expected for each pill – without testing a single patient. All that remained was to complete the deception and to obtain pre-study and post-study electrocardiograms – requested by the drug company – for the non-existent patients. It proved a minor problem, however, for the doctor simply asked a friend to give him copies of normal electrocardiograms taken on patients at the local hospital. He then substituted the names of his fictitious 'guinea pigs' for those of the original patients. Together with the fake medical reports, the electrocardiograms thus appeared to confirm that the drug was totally harmless. [34]

The drug company was so impressed with the doctor's results in this and subsequent studies, that they started sending him to medical conventions. Indeed, they even made a training film in which he

starred. The film was not only used in a medical education programme, but also as advertising in the promotion of the drug.

■In 1980, the Richardson-Merrill Company who we have already
come across in the thalidomide disaster, was sued by Mrs Betty
Mekdeci, the mother of a five-year-old boy with limb and chest
deformities. Mrs Mekdeci claims that the deformities were caused
by Bendectin, an anti-morning sickness pill manufactured by the
company. In Britain the drug is marketed as Debendox.

One of those who testified on behalf of Mrs Mekdeci was Professor William McBride, the Australian obstetrician who first
alerted the world to the dangers of thalidomide. McBride told the
court that he believes the drug is a 'low-grade teratogen'. Although
a jury found for the Mekdecis – awarding them $20,000, a fraction
of the $12 million they were claiming – a federal appeal judge ruled
the verdict unsound and ordered a retrial.

When he returned to Australia after giving evidence at the
trial, Professor McBride discovered that he was under surveillance
by Richardson-Merrill.[35] In August 1980, he received a letter from
Rear-Admiral Gordon Crabb, one-time commander of the Australian fleet. The letter said that Crabb had been approached by a
private investigator acting for Richardson-Merrill, who told him
that the company wanted details of any police or civilian court
proceedings against McBride, and warned that the professor might
be under surveillance.

Since his retirement, Crabb had worked as a consultant on the
prevention of industrial espionage and the private investigator
apparently thought that this was sufficient grounds to rely on him as
an informer. Little did he know the Rear-Admiral. As soon as
Crabb heard the investigator's request, he became incensed. 'I have
told the people concerned,' he wrote to McBride, 'that I do not wish
to be involved in any of their activities.'[36]

In May 1981 a retrial jury ruled that Bendectin had not caused
David Mekdeci's birth defects.[37] The verdict followed an FDA
ruling that there was no demonstrated link between Bendectin and
birth defects.[38] A British report also cleared the drug.[39] In July
1982, however, two controversial animal studies suggested that the
drug could indeed damage the unborn foetus. In the US it was

agreed that a warning label, giving details of the study, should accompany the drug. However, no such action was taken in Britain. [40]

■A 1972 Study by the University of Nebraska Medical School concluded that Flagyl, a vaginal antibiotic which had been on the market for some time, was an outright carcinogen. [41] Hearing of the report, the FDA ordered Dr Adrian Gross of their Scientific Investigations Staff to check the study's data and see if the conclusions were justified. Gross did so and reported that the research did indeed show that Flagyl was a carcinogen. [42] As a result, he went back to the FDA's files and reviewed two studies submitted to the agency by the drug's manufacturer, the Searle Company, which purportedly showed no evidence of carcinogenicity.

'I noticed that there were a number of discrepancies between the raw data and the summary of the raw data submitted by the company,' Gross recalls. 'None of these discrepancies were in any way "alarming" at that particular time; they could have been nothing more than simple typographical errors or mistakes on the part of whoever summarised the raw data. We had no reason to suspect anything more serious.' [43]

Gross was soon to be convinced otherwise. In 1974, Searle submitted an amended version of their original study. 'Among the first things I noticed,' remarks Gross, 'was that in the case of one animal, where in the original report there appeared to be a conflict between the raw data and the summary, in the amended version this discrepancy was no longer present. The way in which this accord was accomplished was that the entry in the *original* report was corrected to agree with the summary.' [44] (Italics added.) Gross also noted that, in the amended version, one animal (a rat in the control group which had not been exposed to Flagyl) had apparently developed a breast tumour – an extremely rare occurrence.

Gross and his colleagues visited Searle's headquarters in May 1974 to examine the original laboratory records for the studies, but was told that the company 'had no records'. [45] He was, however, allowed to examine a slide of the tumour said to be from the male rat that had developed breast cancer. He agreed that the slide did indeed show a tumour, but when he asked for a tissue sample in order to verify that the rat was a male – and not a female fraudulently submitted into the control group – Searle allegedly refused to let him have it. [46]

'I had the sample in my hands,' he recalls, 'but the company forced me to return it to them. When we came back on a subsequent visit and asked for the sample again, they had embodied the entire fixed tissue in paraffin; in other words, they had rendered the tissue unfit for a chromosome sex analysis.' [47] Searle vigorously disputed this. [48]

As a result of the FDA's investigation of Flagyl, the agency decided to look more closely at some of the other tests submitted by Searle. Gross found that studies on Aldactone, a drug to reduce strain and high blood pressure, showed a similar pattern of falsification. In particular, the tests were carried out in such a way that the probability of finding tumours in the animals given the drug was effectively minimised. [49] The same was alleged of a study on Aldactone, carried out by the Hazleton Laboratories under contract to Searle, which Gross describes as 'so questionable, if not outright inadequate or faulty, that a conclusion of "safety" from the carcinogenesis point of view could not have been reached by reasonable reviewers'. [50] Nonetheless, Searle submitted the study as evidence that the drug did not cause cancer.

Although Searle was informed in early 1973 of the results of research undertaken by Microscopy for Biological Research of Albany, New York, which showed a dose-related increase in liver and testicular tumours in rats, the company did not report these findings to the FDA for two years. [51] Indeed, both Hazleton and Searle have been accused of deliberately trying to mislead the FDA's Advisory Committee on Cardiorenal Drugs by playing down the carcinogenic effects of Aldactone. At a meeting in June 1975, during which Searle presented the results of its tests on Aldactone, Dr Weil, a Searle consultant, is said to have shown a statistical table which reported no malignant breast tumours amongst animals exposed to the drug. In fact, there were four such tumours. [52, 53]

There are further instances still in which Searle play an equally suspect role. For example, in support of its application for a licence to market Aspartame, a food sweetener intended to break into the saccharine market, Searle submitted 160 studies to the FDA. Eleven were selected for review and 'numerous problems' were noted.[54] In one instance, a single animal was reported 'alive' and then 'dead' no less than six times.[55] Indeed, even Searle's own consultant felt he could not endorse five of the studies, carried out to test for terato- genic effects. 'Even following the track you did,' he wrote to company officials, 'it seems to me you have only confounded the issue by a series of studies, most of which have severe design deficiencies or obvious lack of expertise in animal management. Because of these twin factors, all the careful and detailed examina- tion of foetuses, all the writing, summarisation and resummarisa- tion is of little avail because of the shaky foundation.'[56]

One of the studies reviewed by the FDA had been carried out by the University of Wisconsin. The study (which tested Aspartame's ability to impair the learning ability of monkeys) was never com- pleted, however, as the researcher died before he could finish final post-medication examinations. According to Dr Schmidt of the FDA: 'In the course of FDA's investigation, questions raised about aspects of the study were repeatedly answered in part with the con- tention that Searle had exercised no control over the study. In fact, Searle files indicate that they initiated contact with the investigator to see if he would carry out such a study and were in frequent contact with him after it began, that they influenced important aspects of its conduct, such as drug dose, that a memorandum calls the study "of first priority with the Searle Company" and paid the investigator $15,000 for being a consultant.' Searle maintained, however, that it was a follow-up study that they had deemed 'of first priority' – a study that was carried on by other researchers after the researcher died.[57]

But perhaps the most interesting document to have emerged from the FDA investigation is a confidential memorandum, headed 'Trade Secrets Information'. Written by company director, Herbert Helling, the memorandum discussed the best tactics to use in order to persuade the FDA to approve Aspartame. It provides an in- triguing insight into boardroom politics:

'These are thoughts on the matter of sweetener stragegy. As I see it, our objective is to obtain approval from the Food and Drug Administration for SC-18852 (Aspartame) for enough uses to permit consumption (and hence production) at a level that will meet the economic requirements. With that in mind, we will say what we need to do, know, or accomplish in order to bring about this objective.

'We must determine which application of the sweetener seems possible and then select from these those that seem most likely to be approved. We must decide what factors Food and Drug would be most concerned about and determine which of these food items would present the least concern (after ranking the concerns in order of our difficulty to meet at this time).

'We should arrange an early informal meeting with Dr Wodicka and Dr Blumenthal. At this meeting, the basic philosophy of our approach to Food and Drug should be to try to get them to say "Yes", to rank the things we are going to ask for so we are putting first those questions we would like to get a "yes" to, even if we have to throw some in that have no significance to us, other than putting them in a "yes" saying habit. We must create an affirmative atmosphere in our dealing with them. It would help if we can get them or their people involved to do us any such favours. This would also help bring them into a subconscious spirit of participation.'[58]

The memorandum goes on to stress that the meetings must be arranged through Dr Wodicka, head of the Bureau of Foods, because he is 'from an industry background and Dr Scott feels he is quite good'. It ends with Helling remarking: 'I think it is very important for us to start to get our sweetener into commercial channels as soon as possible to minimise the incentive that people now have to work on other sweeteners. Actions in the US will tend to influence the actions in other countries as well.'[59] In 1981, Aspartame was approved for marketing in the US after further investigations by the FDA.[60]

■Industrial Biotests Labs (IBT) of Illinois, a subsidiary of the giant Nalco Chemical Company, is one of the largest animal testing laboratories in the USA and has carried out studies on numerous products from drugs to industrial chemicals, food additives and pesticides. In April 1977, after the FDA found that tests on Naprosyn (a widely used anti-arthritis drug) and trichlorocarbon (an antimicrobial agent contained in many brands of soap) had been falsified*, the agency announced that it intended to investigate IBT for 'fraud and submission of questionable test data'.[61] Shortly before the announcement (which was expected for several months), the laboratory shredded its files on thousands of products it had tested previously. A.J. Frisque, the president of the company, admitted giving the order to destroy the documents, but claimed it was due to a 'misunderstanding'.[63]

(Interestingly, Dr Gross warned his director at the FDA's Scientific Investigation Staff in January 1977, of precisely this eventuality: 'Given IBT's track record of not being entirely candid with us, as well as their current embarrassing situation in the FDA and in general throughout the pharmaceutical industry, and given the potential for great economic loss to them if additional "bad news" surfaces, I would not judge it inconceivable that IBT personnel might burn the midnight oil in destroying incriminating data or making up [more favourable] ones, or in general tampering with such records.)[64]

Since it began, the FDA investigation has clearly established that IBT deliberately manipulated a series of carcinogenicity tests and that at least four major pesticide manufacturers participated in the fraud by submitting the studies to government agencies even though they knew they had been falsified.

■An FDA review of 12 studies conducted by Biobasics Laboratories of New York City, found 11 of them to 'have gross discrepancies, ranging from overt fraud to extreme sloppiness'.[65] Investigators also reported that they had difficulty in obtaining records of some of the studies. In one instance, the office of a doctor they wished to interview was vandalised the night before their inspection

---

* Of the Naprosyn study, Dr Gross wrote: 'It is my personal conviction that in the reports submitted to the FDA, IBT both withheld material information and substituted false information either of which could have affected our view. In my own mind the evidence for this is overwhelming.' His criticism of the trichlorocarbon study is equally severe, and he notes that the manufacturers, Monsanto, 'is certainly not presenting a thorough searching and critical report of their own audit (if any) of IBT's records.'[62]

was due. Dr Hensley, medical officer of the FDA's Scientific Investigation Staff, described the incident to the 1979 Kennedy Committee:

'The sofas were cut up; reverse swastikas were painted on the walls. It was interesting that it appeared that the [doctor's] certificates and diplomas had been removed from the walls before the swastikas were painted. The outlines were clearly visible where they had hung, as well as the nails. The records relating to the studies that we were going to look at, together with some other patients' records, had been dumped into a whirlpool bath and turned on overnight. Of course, we had to postpone the investigation while the police made their reports. We rescheduled for a date a couple of weeks later. In the interim, there was a fire that started mysteriously in the doctor's office. Apparently, a stack of paper towels in the middle of the floor of the back-room, next to the record room, caught fire spontaneously.' [66]

Eventually, the FDA managed to get hold of the relevant documents and found that there was little evidence that the doctor had ever carried out the five studies he claimed he had undertaken. Indeed, when patients who were supposed to have participated in the studies were interviewed, all denied any knowledge of them.

■In August 1982, sales of the anti-arthritic drug, Opren, were 'suspended' in Britain after the Committee on the Safety of Medicines received complaints from doctors that the drug caused bizarre side effects, including the regrowth of hair in bald men, the growth of facial hair in women and the acceleration of the growth rate of finger and toe nails. Sixty-one people were thought to have died as a result of taking this drug. The Committee on the Safety of Medicines, which had taken eight months to act over the drug, is still (at the time of writing) reviewing Opren's record. In America the drug was also withdrawn amid allegations that the manufacturers, Eli Lilly, had withheld the results of clinical tests which showed adverse side effects. It is uncertain whether or not the drug will be permitted back on the market.

Shortly before this edition of Cover-Up went to press full

details of the Opren affair were revealed in a two-part documentary by Tom Mangold of the BBC Panorama programme.

The cases described above are just a handful of those which have come to light in recent years. Undoubtedly, many more remain firmly locked in company files. Certainly, investigators allege numerous other incidents, but without documentary proof they are unable to substantiate their allegations. When that proof is unearthed, the degree to which even top management is involved in decisions which they know will cost lives, is often shocking.

In the meantime, the public continues to take prescribed drugs on the assumption that manufacturers have the general health of the population at heart. How much longer will it be before the true facts emerge?

8
ASBESTOS: THE SLOW KILLER

ASBESTOS IS just one of the thousands of toxic substances to which industrial workers are exposed. Few of those substances have been tested for likely ill effects, and their continued use has resulted in a rapid increase in the number of workers succumbing to crippling occupational diseases. When the dangers *are* discovered, the relevant industries often find their very existence threatened – a motive for keeping the workers and the public in the dark is clear. In the case of asbestos, that cover-up resulted from a decision taken at the very highest boardroom level in numerous international corporations. It has lasted for some fifty years.

It took a chance discovery by Karl Asch, a lawyer representing victims of asbestosis and cancer, to explode the deception.

Under American law, before a case comes to court the parties in a lawsuit are permitted a discovery period during which they are expected to collect evidence to support their case: sworn 'depositions' are taken from key witnesses and relevant documents are obtained if necessary by subpoena. It was during such a discovery period that Asch came across an extraordinary cache of letters. He was investigating a compensation claim on behalf of an asbestos insulation worker who had developed lung cancer. As part of that investigation, Asch spent three days questioning the president of Raybestos-Manhatten, the company being sued and one of the largest manufacturers of asbestos products in the United States. During the interview, he noticed a dusty cardboard box on a shelf in a cupboard. When he asked what the box contained, he was told that it was full of old company files. Asch rummaged through them and was astonished by what he found. Dubbed the 'Asbestos Pentagon Papers' by the press, the files revealed a concerted and deliberate attempt by the asbestos industry to suppress any research that might dent its sales or undermine its official position that asbestos manufacturers could not be held liable for asbestos-related disease among those using their products. It was truly an extraordinary record . . .

Asbestos is an extraordinary mineral. A silicate compound, it is mined in much the same way as tin or iron. Unlike those minerals, however, asbestos is made up of fibres – ranging in length from a millionth of an inch to over a foot – which can be separated out and spun into a fabric*. Once woven, the 'cloth' is used in such diverse products as brake linings, roof insulation, oven linings, blankets and clothing, air filters and fire doors. Not that its unique properties are a modern discovery. It is probable that its ability to resist heat has been known for thousands of years; certainly the archaeological record suggests that some 4,000 years ago Finnish potters mixed asbestos fibres in the clay to make their cooking pots.[2] And the ancient Greek and Roman nobility valued the quality of the woven cloth so highly that it was fashionable to be buried in shrouds manufactured from it.[3]

Unfortunately, it is asbestos's unique feature of separating into fibres that makes it such a potent health hazard. For, released into the air, those fibres form a dust which if inhaled can cause irreparable damage. Once lodged in the lungs, the fibres lacerate the delicate tissues of the bronchial tubes, causing hard and thick scars to develop. In time – and it takes a minimum of ten years for the symptoms to appear – the scarring can cause cancer, or asbestosis, a crippling respiratory disease which (although not always fatal in itself) leads to breathlessness and severe chest pains after the slightest physical effort.

---

* Spun asbestos's fibrous quality has led to much confusion. As Dr Alan Dalton writes in his book, *Asbestos: Killer Dust*: 'Because it is fibrous, many people think it is a plant product like cotton or rope: in fact, as recently as the 1960s, a major share-holder in an asbestos company, visiting the source of his supplier in South Africa, asked his manager where the plantations were.'[1]

In the final stages of the disease, asbestosis victims cannot even climb up stairs without having to rest on each step. Death normally results from a massive heart attack caused by the sheer strain of pumping blood through the damaged lungs.

The first case of asbestosis was diagnosed by a British doctor, Montague Murray, in 1906.[4]* Although Murray reported his findings to the government's Enquiry on Compensation, he evidently did not consider the disease of sufficient importance to publish details of the case in any medical journal. Indeed, it was not until 1924 – by which time US insurance companies were refusing to sell life insurance policies to asbestos workers – that the disease was first described clinically in the medical literature. That report, written by W.E. Cooke for the *British Medical Journal*,[5] was followed by a spate of studies (predominantly from British researchers) documenting the high incidence of the disease among textile workers employed weaving asbestos fibres. Prompted by these reports, the British Factory Inspectorate conducted a survey of workers in the asbestos industry and found asbestosis in one-third of all those employed for more than five years.[6] As a result, in 1933 the British government introduced legislation to reduce occupational exposure of workers to asbestos dust. Asbestosis was also made a compensational disease.

Although the Factory Inspectorate's report and the new British safety standards were published in the American *Journal of Industrial Hygiene*,[7] the US asbestos industry resolutely opposed any attempts to introduce similar regulations into the United States. That stance was maintained throughout the forties and fifties, even in the face of studies showing that 13 per cent of those dying from asbestosis had lung cancer; that asbestosis gets worse even when the victim is removed from the source of asbestos dust; and that those working with asbestos had ten times the risk of dying from lung cancer.[8] Indeed, it was not until 1964 – after Professor Irving Selikoff of Mount Sinai Medical School, New York, published a study showing that asbestos insulation workers had a greater chance of dying from lung disease than the average white male[9] – that the US asbestos industry reluctantly began to place warning labels on its products.†About the

---

* Murray diagnosed the first case in modern times. The Romans were well aware of asbestosis.

† See over.

same time as Selikoff's findings were published, reports began to dribble out of South Africa and British shipyards that 7 to 8 per cent of asbestos workers – 1,000 times the numbers expected – were dying from mesothelioma, a rare cancer of the cells lining the chest and abdominal cavities. [11]

Selikoff, who was denied access to industry data on asebstos workers' health, had carried out his study on 632 members of the International Association of Heat and Frost Insulation and Asbestos Workers. He has continued to follow their fate. By 1977, he found 478 of the original group had died – one fifth of them from lung cancer. [12] Indeed, the number of lung cancer cases exceeded the number expected in a normal population by a factor of seven. [13] Selikoff also notes that the rates of stomach, colon and rectum cancers were three times that expected – hardly surprising, perhaps, for as Selikoff points out: 'Anyone who inhales dust also tends to ingest it.' [14]

Until Selikoff's 1964 study, the asbestos manufacturers maintained that there was insufficient evidence to justify a warning label and that, being unaware of the health hazard, they could not be held liable for injuries to those who had used their products prior to that date. The letters found by Asch in Raybestos-Manhattan's head office exploded that defence once and for all. Indeed, when they were shown to South Carolina circuit judge, James Price, he was so shocked by what he termed 'this pattern of denial and attempts at suppression of information' that he ordered a retrial of a compensation case on a dead insulation worker. [15]

In 1929, Dr Anthony Lanza of the Metropolitan Life Insurance Company was commissioned to undertake a survey of the health of randomly selected asbestos workers with more than three years of employment. The study, which showed that 53 per cent of the workers had asbestosis, was completed in 1931, but was not published until 1935. [16] Before publication, Lanza dutifully sent galley proofs to Johns-Manville, the world's largest asbestos producer, and Raybestos-Manhattan, both of whom had sponsored his research. The galleys were forwarded to Johns-Manville's lawyer, George Hobart, who

---

† Johns-Manville, the world's largest asbestos producer, was first to do so in 1964. Raybestos-Manhattan, on the other hand, delayed until 1972 when labels became mandatory. [10]

noted that several of Lanza's comments might effectively undermine the company's principal defence in any future negligence suits – namely that too little was known about asbestosis to hold the owners of asbestos plants responsible for failing to take proper precautions to protect their workers from the disease. Hobart was particularly concerned about one sentence in the report which likened asbestosis to silicosis, a lung disease caused by inhaling silica dust. His concern was understandable, for the State Legislature of New Jersey, where Johns-Manville had its main factory, was about to recognise silicosis as a compensable disease.[17] Any acknowledgement by the industry that asbestosis was similar to silicosis could easily result in asbestosis also being recognised. 'It would be very helpful to have an official report to show that there is a substantial difference between asbestosis and silicosis, and, by the same token, it would be troublesome if an official report should appear from which the conclusion might be drawn that there is very little, if any, difference between the two diseases.'[18] Hobart went on to endorse a suggestion by Johns-Manville's chief attorney, Vandiver Brown, that Lanza should reinsert a sentence he had deleted from his original report. The sentence read: 'Clinically, from this study, asbestosis appeared to be a type of disease milder than silicosis.'

Hobart's comments, together with several other suggestions for changes in the text of the report, were sent to Lanza by Vandiver Brown with a covering letter. 'I am sure you will understand fully that no one in our organisation is suggesting for a moment that you alter by one jot or title any scientific facts or inevitable conclusions revealed or justified by your preliminary survey,' he wrote. 'All we ask is that all of the favourable aspects of the survey be included and that none of the unfavourable be unintentionally pictured in darker tones than the circumstances justify. I feel confident that we can depend upon you and Dr McConnell to give us this "break", and mine and Mr Hobart's suggestions are presented in this spirit.'[19] Apparently, Lanza felt able to play ball, for the final sentence Brown and Hobart had urged him to reinstate was included word for word in the final published text, as were other suggested changes. In any event, the study had its desired effect: asbestosis was not recognised as a compensable disease in New Jersey until 1945.[20]

Not that Johns-Manville refused point-blank to compensate

workers. Rather, the company did not want the settlements put on a statutory basis. Minutes of two meetings in 1933 reveal that the company's board voted to settle eleven asbestos cases, due to be heard in a New Jersey court, for $30,000. The settlement, however, was conditional of a written assurance being obtained 'from the attorney for the various plaintiffs that he would not directly or indirectly participate in the bringing of new actions against the corporation'.[21]

The letters found by Asch also include a revealing correspondence between the editor of the trade magazine, *Asbestos*, and Sumner Simpson, the president of Raybestos-Manhattan. Following a decision by the New York Legislature to make asbestosis compensable, the magazine wrote to the company asking for permission to publish an article on the disease and on modern methods of dust control. Even by the deferential standards of the 1930s, the phrasing of the request is remarkable:

> 'You may recall that we have written to you on several occasions concerning the publishing of information, or discussion of asbestosis and the work which has been done, or is being done, to eliminate or at least reduce it.
>
> 'Always you have requested that for certain obvious reasons we publish nothing, and naturally your wishes have been respected.
>
> 'Possibly by this time, however, the reasons for your objection to publicity on this subject have been eliminated, and if so, we would very much like to review the whole matter in *Asbestos* . . .
>
> 'We await with much interest your reply. If there is no serious objection it would seem to be a most interesting subject for the pages of *Asbestos*, and possibly with a discussion of it in *Asbestos* along the right lines, would serve to combat some of the rather undesirable publicity given to it in current newspapers.'[22]

Simpson sent the letter to Vandiver Brown, with the comment: 'As I see it personally, we would be just as well off to say nothing about it until our survey is complete. I think the less said about asbestos the better off we are, but at the same time, we cannot lose track of the fact that there have been a number of articles on asbestos dust controls and asbestosis in the British trade magazines. The magazine *Asbestos* is in business to publish articles affecting the trade and they have been very decent about not reprinting the English articles.'[23] Brown replied: 'I quite agree with you that our interests are best served by having asbestosis receive a minimum of publicity.'[24]

By 1936, with adverse reports of asbestosis stacking up, Simpson wrote to five other companies, suggesting they might like to participate in funding a study on the effects of asbestos on rats. Simpson made it quite clear that the research could do no harm as it would be totally under the companies' control. 'From time to time, after the findings are made we can determine whether we wish any publication or not,' he wrote. 'My own view is that it would be a good thing to distribute the information among the medical fraternity, providing it is of the right type and would not injure our companies.'[25]

The research was duly funded and carried out at the Saranac Laboratories, New York, by Dr Leroy Gardner, whose contract stipulated that 'the results of these studies shall become the property of the (contributing companies) and the manuscripts of any reports shall be submitted for approval of the contributors before publication'.[26] Recently discovered documents show that Gardner found a high incidence of lung cancer in mice exposed to both long and short fibres – findings which he reported to both Vandiver Brown and other sponsors in a draft monograph on asbestosis. The monograph, however, was not published and Gardner died three years later in 1946.[27]

Although the medical director of Johns-Manville, Dr Kenneth Smith, knew from X-rays taken in 1948 that workers at one of the company's Canadian plants were suffering from asbestosis – but had not yet developed its crippling symptoms – he recommended that they should not be told of their illness. 'The fibrosis is irreversible and permanent so that eventually compensation will be paid to each of these men,' he wrote in a confidential memorandum. 'But as long as the man is not disabled it is felt that he should not be told of his condition so that he can live and work in peace and the company can benefit by his many years of experience. Should the man be told of his conditions there is a very definite probability that he would become mentally and physically ill simply through the knowledge that he had asbestosis.'[28] However, Smith did recommend that the company place warning labels on their products – a recommendation that was turned down. A Johns-Manville plant manager recently testified that the company had a policy of not informing workers if their medical check-ups showed signs of asbestosis right up until 1971.[29]

In 1952, the Industrial Hygiene Foundation (described by Vandiver Brown as 'a creature of industry and an institution upon which employers can rely for a completely sympathetic approach to their viewpoint')[30] proposed that the US Asbestos Textile Institute conduct a cancer survey among its workers. The proposal was rejected, after a similar study in Britain showed a high rate of lung cancer, for fear 'that such an investigation would stir up a hornets' nest and put the whole industry under suspicion'.[31] Although a study was eventually undertaken, it was described by Dr Wilhelm Hueper, the founding father of the science of epidemiology, as 'statistical acrobatics which tend to obscure incriminating evidence'.[32]

Two years before Selikoff produced his study of New York insulation workers, the Philip-Carey Manufacturing Company hired Dr Thomas Mancuso to conduct a study of the health of workers in one of its factories. It was hoped that 'from the claims standpoint, Dr Mancuso, as a nationally credited expert, can help to differentiate an expensive asbestosis or silicosis case from non-occupational illnesses, such as cancer or bronchitis, and make the defence stand up'.[33] The company had evidently misjudged Mancuso, a man of the highest integrity, who was not going to tailor his conclusions simply because the company was paying for his services. After finding an excess rate of cancer, he published the results in 1963 and, in a confidential report, urged the company to clean up their plant and warn consumers of the dangers asbestos posed to their health. Philip-Carey, now taken over by Celotex, did not do so until 1971. Mancuso told me that they deny receiving his recommended safety improvements.[34]

The controversy over appropriate warning labels for asbestos products did not stop with the US government's 1972 decision to make them mandatory. In 1977, the European Commission published a damning report, 'Public Health Risks of Exposure to Asbestos',[35] warning that no level of exposure to asbestos could be considered safe and urging that measures be introduced immediately to reduce dust levels to the lowest practicable limit. In the wake of the report, European manufacturers found themselves under enormous pressure to strengthen their warning labels. [36]

Meanwhile, the lines were being drawn for yet another battle. In 1972, the US Occupational Safety and Health Administration reacted to the growing evidence of lung disease amongst asbestos workers by reducing occupational exposure to 2 million fibres per cubic metre of air – a standard which had been in force in Britain since 1968. That standard was based on a report by the British Occupational Hygiene Society (BOHS). Yet, as Alan Dalton of the British Society of Social Responsibility in Science points out, five of the nine members of the BOHS's asbestos sub-committee were actually employed by the asbestos industry: and the single medical study on which the 2 fibre standard was set was later found to be seriously flawed. [37] The study had been carried out by Turner and Newall, Britain's largest asbestos manufacturers, at its Rochdale plant and allegedly found asbestosis in only 3 per cent of the 290 workers it examined. In 1969, however, Dr Knox, the company doctor who had supervised the study, was replaced by Dr Hilton Lewinsohn, who subsequently re-examined the 290 workers. He found signs of asbestosis in 50 per cent of the workers. [38]

By 1980, the 2 fibre standard was under attack as grossly inadequate. A major problem was that standard monitoring techniques could only detect asbestos fibres over 5 microns in length. Yet electron microscopes reveal that for every long fibre detected, hundreds of smaller ones go uncounted. From then on arithmetic takes over: a man, inhaling an estimated 8 cubic metres of air in an average working day, will be seen to be breathing in only 16 million fibres – assuming that dust levels are kept within the limits. In fact, as Samual Epstein points out, he may be inhaling as many as 1.6 billion short fibres. [39] Moreover, laboratory studies reveal that it is those fine undetected asbestos fibres which pose the greatest danger to human health. Indeed, in 1976 the US National Institute of Occupational Safety and Health was alarmed enough by the evidence to propose a twentyfold reduction in the US standard to 100,000 fibres per cubic metre. In defence of that reduction, NIOSH cited studies which showed that workers exposed to 250,000 fibres had twice the expected rate of asbestosis and lung cancer. [40]

In 1982, the British Health and Safety Commission announced that it was to cut the permitted 2 fibre standard for asbestos dust to 1 fibre per cubic centimetre – a level which has been described as 'arbitrary'.[41] The asbestos industry – which largely operates at the 1 fibre standard already – opposed moves to cut the permissible level to 0.5 fibres.[42, 43] The cut, however, has not been made without a fight by the asbestos industry – including a £500,000 public relations campaign. That campaign was described at the time as being part of a general campaign 'to "influence reports, legislation and government recommendations on new safety standards".'[44]

Some of the statements made during that campaign, whilst not actually untrue, tell only half the story. It was claimed in a full-page advertisement in the national dailies, for example, that 'the risks of getting an asbestos disease are almost always confined to those who worked with asbestos some years ago – before present safety regulations were introduced. Asbestos only becomes dangerous when the dust is breathed in excessive amounts, generally over a long period'.[45] What the advertisement omits to say, however, is that asbestosis had been found amongst many wives of asbestos workers who breathed in the dust whilst cleaning their husbands' overalls, and also amongst those living near (but not working in) asbestos mines and mills.[46] Either asbestos can, as experts at both NIOSH and the European Commission claim, cause lung diseases at extremely low levels of exposure or we must assume that those cases resulted from excessive exposure over a long period. In which case, what are we to make of the advertisements' claim that asbestos levels in the atmosphere 'indicate no health hazard to the general public'? Are asbestos workers' wives and those who live near asbestos mines and mills no longer members of the 'general public'?

In fact, one US expert, Benjamin Suta of the Stanford Research Institute, has warned that 'asbestos exposures for non-occupationally exposed people can, at times, match or exceed exposures for people employed in asbestos professions'.[47] He points out that a quarter to a half of those living in major US cities have been found to have asbestos particles in their lungs; and that virtually all of us are now exposed to asbestos in the water we drink and the food we eat – particularly processed foods. As Lawrence McGinty of *New Scientist* remarks somewhat sardonically: 'Although asbestos is far from the most potent toxic substance used industrially, its very pervasiveness means that the number of people exposed to it – workers, consumers, and those living in cities – is enormous. It would be quicker to count those who haven't been exposed.'[48]

Official estimates in the United States put the potential death toll from asbestos exposure amongst workers alone at 2 million. In Britain it is possible that some 500,000 workers will die from asbestos related diseases over the next thirty years. If that proves the case then, as Alan Dalton of the British Society for Social Responsibility in Science remarks: 'Asbestos exposure will kill more people in Britain than were killed in the armed forces during the Second World War.'[49]

Faced with a sky-rocketing bill for compensation claims, the US asbestos industry is now fighting a desperate last ditch battle to survive. 'John McKinney, the chairman of Johns-Manville, is coping with an avalanche of litigation from workers who were exposed to his company's products,' reports Stephen Solomon in *Fortune* magazine. 'He spends half of his time on the asbestos problem, directing the company's strategy and meeting with legislators and security analysts. The company has had trouble on both Capitol Hill and on Wall Street. During a series of Congressional hearings on asbestos (in August 1978) the price of Johns-Manville stocks plunged about 20 per cent.'[50]

By July 1981, more than 400 new compensation claims were being filed every month against Johns-Manville – one every 30 minutes of every working day. A year later, facing some 16,500 law suits, Johns-Manville filed for bankruptcy, thus freezing all future litigation but allowing the company to continue trading.[51] At the time, it was estimated by Lloyd's of London that asbestosis suits had cost the world's insurance industry some £58,000 million.[52, 53]

The news of Johns-Manville's bankruptcy came hard on the heels of a Yorkshire Television programme which alleged that Britain's largest asbestos company, Turner and Newall, had misled a government inquiry about the incidence of asbestosis. According to Yorkshire Television: 'Turner's told the asbestos inquiry in 1977 that the prevalence of asbestos-disease in their British factories was no more than 1 in 300. Yet Dr John Morris, then Turner's chief medical officer and a former University lecturer, was within a few months of concluding that the number of definite or strongly suspected cases of asbestosis at Turner's Rochdale (plant) was not 1 in 300 but more than 1 in 4. The main asbestos inquiry authors never received Dr

Morris's vital 1 in 4 findings from Turner's and they were never published.'[54]

Turned and Newall rigorously denied the charges made by Yorkshire Television: in a press statement, the company said that none of its companies had 'knowingly supplied false information nor (had) any information been suppressed on the subject of asbestos and health.'[55] In answer to a question from the General and Municipal Workers' Union, however, the company admitted that a statement it had made in 1978 – that the death rate from lung cancer at its Rochdale factory did not 'differ significantly from the national average' – was 'incorrect'. The statement, said the company 'should have been qualified to refer to our experience to date in respect of low dust levels in the weaving department since 1951'.[56] The weaving department employs 135 out of the 800-odd workers at the plant. In 1977, a study by an Oxford researcher estimated that the total lung cancer rate at the plant was twice the expected rate for the general population.[57] Following the television programme, Turner and Newall – which expected to pay out £6.6 million in 1982 in compensation claims – saw its shares fall by 14 per cent in just one day.[58]

Meanwhile, the asbestos industry has begun to 'export' its factories to the Third World where pollution laws are few and far between and compensation claims are not the problems they are in the West. 'In 1972', reports Barry Castleman, an environmental consultant, 'Amatex, a firm based in Norristown, Pennsylvania, closed a new (opened in 1967) asbestos yarn factory in Milford Square, Pennsylvania. Since 1969, Amatex has operated an asbestos textile plant in Agua Prieta, a small town just across the Mexican border from Douglas, Arizona.'[59] Conditions at the plant were appalling: in 1977, a journalist on the *Arizona Daily Star* described how asbestos was strewn across access roads to the plant; how waste clung to the boundary fence and littered the machinery in the weaving plant; and how many workers did not wear protective masks.[60] Even after the owners cleaned up the factory, a distinguished industrial health specialist was to describe the improvements as 'cosmetic'.[61]

There is growing concern, too, about health and safety practices at other foreign-owned asbestos factories in the Third World. In 1980, for instance, a former employee of Hindustan Ferodo Ltd. of India alleged that workers at the company's Bombay factory were not told 'at all' about the dangers of asbestos; that the plant's products were not labelled as to possible health risks; and that workers were not informed about the results of medical checks.[62] The company – in which Turner and Newall had a 74 per cent holding – denied the allegations.[63] In 1982, Turner and Newall became involved in another controversy after the *Observer* published the results of a study by the UK Medical Research Council which had found extremely high dust levels in an asbestos mine and mill owned by a subsidiary of the company at Havelock in Swaziland.[64] In some parts of the mill, the dust levels were as high as 50 fibres per cubic centimetre – 25 times the British 2 fibre safety standard. The levels, measured in 1976, have since been reduced – in line with a 1976 commitment 'to apply the current British safety standard in our factories throughout the world'. In August 1982, the 'average personal exposure' for the 2,100 workers at Havelock was, according to a company spokesman, below the 2 fibre standard: nonetheless, '4 per cent of the workforce' were still receiving 'the equivalent of between two and three fibres'.[65] If the British standards were not yet in force at Havelock, said Mr H. Hardie, personnel director of Turner and Newall, in an answer to the *Observer* article (which he called 'misleading'), it was because 'sadly, the implementation of policy can take time'.[66]

Undoubtedly the Third World will increasingly become a haven for asbestos manufacturers. Anxious for foreign exchange, Third World governments have already bent over backwards to give investing companies a free rein, even at the expense of the health and safety of the local population. Such callous disregard for human life is appalling enough when perpetrated in ignorance. When the dangers have been known for decades, it is totally inexcusable.

9
LEAD:
THE POISON IN OUR PETROL

LEAD HAS been called Britain's number one pollutant.[1] It may not be the most toxic, but it is certainly one of the most widespread. Due largely to the practice of adding it to our petrol, motor exhaust ensures that we are all at risk. That practice, banned in several countries, has repeatedly been declared safe by the British government. Yet the evidence tells a different story – and alarmingly it is our children who are most likely to suffer from the wilful conspiracy to keep the public in the dark.

'I encountered abuse of a kind that I have never encountered anywhere in my life before, in social or academic circles. It is an experience I shall never forget. I will not be prepared to serve on any government working party again after this . . .'[2] Dr Robert Stephens was talking after being viciously attacked by civil servants from the Department of the Environment for questioning their smooth assurances that lead pollution from car exhausts could not cause brain damage to children. Stephens, a member of the DOE's working party which examined lead levels around Spaghetti Junction in Birmingham, was alarmed by reports that lead levels in the milk teeth of children living in the area between 1973 and 1976 ranged between 0.8 and 108 parts per million (ppm) – the average being 11.8 ppm.[3] Studies from America and elsewhere had already revealed that such levels of lead could cause mental retardation and behavioural defects – and Stephens estimated that, on the basis of the figures obtained by the working party, no less than 20 per cent of the children in Birmingham's inner city area were likely to be suffering from damage to the central nervous system.[4] That estimate conflicted directly with the working party's own reassuring conclusion that there was no cause for alarm over lead pollution levels from traffic using Spaghetti Junction.[5] Hence the civil servants' angry reaction.[6]

Between 7,500 and 10,000 tonnes of lead are pumped into our atmosphere each year – 90 per cent of which comes from petrol fumes.[7] Lead is added to petrol to prevent 'engine knocking', although ironically it actually harms the engine by causing exhaust valve erosion, spark plug erosion, piston ring sticking and lead deposits in the oil.[8] Due to concerns over health hazards, leaded petrol has been banned in Russia and Japan for some years and is currently being phased out in Sweden, America and Australia. The British government, however, is adamant that its present controls are sufficient to protect the British public – a position that is now strongly criticised by numerous independent scientists.

The fumes from car exhausts are contaminated with tetra-ethyl lead (TEL) a compound so dangerous that it is not available for sale on the open market.[9] Indeed, even university researchers have difficulty in obtaining it.[10] Yet, as Anthony Tucker points out in his book, *The Toxic Metals*, every mile that the average saloon car travels, 50 milligrams of this lethal substance is pumped into the atmosphere.[11] 'You can only excrete half a milligram of lead a day and, even with intakes well below that level, lead slowly builds up in tissue and bone. Further, although most of the lead alkyls in fuel are converted into inorganic compounds during combustion, a proportion of the lead coming out of a tailpipe is still in its alkyl form, an even more insidious and deadly poison than any of the inorganic forms. . . the body itself turns tetra-alkyl lead into a deadly brain poison.'[12]

The controversy over the power of lead to cause brain damage is nothing new. As early as 1964, Dr A.A. Moncrieff and his colleagues at Great Ormond Street Hospital, London, found what appeared to be a convincing link between lead pollution and lowered intelligence.[13] Out of 122 mentally retarded or psychologically disturbed children between 6 months and 14 years of age, 45 per cent (55 children) had more than 36 micrograms/100 millilitres (μg/100 ml) of lead in their blood. 12 out of 40 children suffering from encephalitis – an inflammation of the brain – and 28 out of 52 children suffering from abdominal pains, vomiting and general irritability also has blood-lead levels greater than 36 μg/100 ml. [14] Moncrieff and his colleagues concluded that blood-lead levels between 40-60 μg/100 ml should be regarded as potentially dangerous and warned that 'a change in behaviour may be associated with lead toxicity'. [15] They also recommended that a 'safe' threshold – the hypothetical point below which exposure to a toxin is judged to cause no biological damage – for children should be a blood-level of 0.36 μg/100 ml. [16] Nonetheless, they later denied that lead was the primary cause of the childrens' disorders – this despite evidence they themselves presented that one little girl who underwent 'deleading' treatment with penicillamine became 'easier to handle, more alert and more interested in her surroundings'. [17]

Significantly, the very same year that Moncrieff and his fellow researchers at Great Ormond Street clarified their earlier findings, a study of 73 children in Manchester showed that some 20 per cent of those examined had blood-lead levels which exceeded 50 μg/100 ml. Almost 30 per cent exceeded the 36 μg/100 ml 'safety' threshold recommended by Moncrieff. [18] Eleven years later, the blood-lead levels of pre-school children in Birmingham were found to range as high as 89 μg/100 ml. [19]

Since Moncrieff's study, a growing body of evidence has been built up showing that even low levels of lead can cause brain damage. In 1977, researchers at McGill University, Montreal, found that 'learning disabled' children had 5-6 times higher levels of lead in their hair – an indicator of past exposure to lead – than a normal control group. [20] Meanwhile, in 1978, Dr G. Winneke of the *Institut für Lufthygiene und Silikoseforschung*, Düsseldorf found that children with only 7 to 13 ppm of lead in their teeth – another good indicator of past expsoure – fared significantly less well in IQ tests than children with lower lead levels. [21] On the basis of that study, the IQ ratings of over 76 per cent of children in Birmingham (where average tooth-lead levels in children are 11.8 ppm) could be affected. [22]

Earlier, in animal experiments, Winneke had noted that rats with modestly elevated blood-lead levels 20-30 (μg/100 ml) fared less well in intelligence tests than a control group with lower blood-lead levels of less than 0.03 ppm. [23] Significantly, Winneke found that when it came to learning simple tasks, both groups of rats competed equally against each other: when, however, it came to learning more complex tasks (involving, for instance, a degree of visual discrimination) the rats with elevated blood-lead levels were unable to cope as well as the control group. [24] That finding suggests that lead may well cause the greatest damage to the *highest* centres of the brain, allowing victims to go about their daily tasks but diminishing their powers of complex thought. [25]

Winneke's 1978 study had been carried out on a relatively small group of children. Later that same year, a much larger American study confirmed his results. The study had been undertaken by Dr Herbert Needleman, a psychiatrist then at Harvard but now at Pittsburg University. [26] Needleman had analysed the tooth-lead levels of over 2,000 'normal' Boston schoolchildren and correlated those levels with the childrens' general behaviour. In a series of experiments, measuring a broad range of 'mental functions', he tested the childrens' ability to follow simple directions and to carry out a sequence of commands, their reaction times, their hearing, their powers of language and their IQs. In addition, he asked the childrens' teachers to report on their classroom behaviour, assessing the degree to which they might be classified as 'disturbed' through such indicators as their proneness to hyperactivity and the extent to which they displayed signs of frustration, impulsiveness and irritability. [27]

Needleman found that those children with elevated lead-tooth levels faired consistently worse in the mental function tests than those with low lead levels. Indeed, as Des Wilson, Director of CLEAR (the Campaign for Lead-Free Air) reports: 'An IQ deficit of 4-5 points was demonstrated between the high and the low lead group, a deficit which could not be explained away on the basis of any of the other 39 variables analysed in the study.* No child with high lead levels had an

---

* With regard to Needleman's analysis of those other 'variables' which might have accounted for the observed differences in mental ability and behaviour between the high-lead and low-lead groups, Professor Bryce-Smith and his colleagues on the Conservation Society's Pollution Working Party comment: 'One of the most impressive features of Needleman's comparison of matched groups was the great attention given to a total of 39 sociological, medical, and other non-lead factors which might have affected the subject's development and behaviour. Statistical analysis of variance showed that none of these factors could account for the observed differences between the high- and low-lead children. A conclusion which appears to follow from this, though it was not drawn by Needleman, is that lead burdens are not to be seen as merely one among a host of social and other factors

IQ greater than 125, whereas 5 per cent of low lead level children exceeded this level. At the other end of the scale, no child with a low lead level had an IQ less than 72, whereas 5 per cent of the high lead children had IQs of less than 66.'[29]

Needleman also found that a child's classroom behaviour showed a *direct* 'dose-response' relationship to the concentration of lead in his or her teeth – incidents of disturbed behaviour (and this applied to all the indices measured by Needleman) rising in step with increases in tooth lead levels. Lead levels in the children ranged from below 5.1 ppm to above 27.0 ppm – a range considered normal in children today. Significantly Needleman was unable to find a 'threshold' below which there were no effects.[30]

Needleman's study caused a furore in academic circles. Hardly surprising, since according to Nick Kollerstrom, a former researcher at the Air Pollution Research Unit of the Medical Research Council and author of the excellent book, *Lead on the Brain*, Needleman's work 'dispelled the miasma of uncertainty' from the whole question of the effects of lead on the intelligence and behaviour of children.[31] Subsequent studies in other countries have broadly confirmed Needleman's results – and in some cases led to political action in order to reduce the lead content of petrol. In 1979, the State of New South Wales, Australia, opted to make lead-free petrol available and to go lead-free by 1980. That decision – now taken up by the Australian Government – followed a report by researchers at the University of New South Wales which found that lead caused symptoms of brain damage and mental retardation at blood-lead levels of 25 μg/100 ml (0.25 ppm).[32] One fifth of children in the State were estimated to have blood-lead levels above this level – 'an alarming situation of epidemic proportions'.[33] As to the source of the lead, the scientists at the New South Wales University had no illusion: airborne lead, they said, was to blame and motor vehicles were the primary cause for putting lead into the atmosphere.[34]

Whilst Australia acted, however, Britain buried its head in the

---

which influence the development of a normal child's brain and personality, but rather *the* most important single factor yet discovered. That, if true, carries far-reaching implications. Nevertheless, the relationship between neurochemistry and behaviour is a two-way affair: changed neurochemistry alters behaviour, and altered behaviour changes neurochemistry.'[28]

sands. In 1980, an official government working party, under the chairmanship of Professor Patrick Lawther of St Bartholomews Hospital, assured the British public that it had 'seen no firm evidence that lead from petrol has caused harm'.[35] Others were less sanguine. Indeed, many in the environmental movement were sorely disappointed by the report, *Lead and Health*, maintaining that the working party had glossed over evidence they considered vital.

'Although three pages (of the report) were devoted to Indian medicines and cosmetics,'* comments Nick Kollerstrom, 'other aspects of the situation received less thorough treatment. No mention was made of the highly neurotoxic properties of TEL . . . no animal experiments were discussed, such as Winneke's vitally important work, even though it is standard practice in establishing toxicological criteria to proceed by means of such animal experiments . . . The 1979 New South Wales report was described as if it were purely a survey of blood-lead levels amongst Sydney schoolchildren and nothing more. Its investigation into learning difficulties, ill-health and anti-social behaviour in relation to these levels was simply not mentioned. DHSS ministers, who claim to be taking the Lawther report as a basis for policy, will derive from it no information as to why, following the publication of the Sydney Schoolchildren report, the continent of Australia decided to go lead-free as soon as possible.'[36] Indeed to many in the anti-lead lobby (and to others too), the report seemed, at best, to be little more than a whitewash job – and a rather crude one at that.

The Lawther Committee's treatment of Needleman's work is indicative of the whole tone of its report. After devoting considerable space to the Boston Study, the working party dismissed its conclusions on the grounds that pica – a habit found amongst some children for chewing old paint (which contains lead) from old buildings – could explain Needleman's results.†[37] In fact, Needleman had dealt fully

---

* These contain lead. Hair colouring products may contain up to 3 per cent lead.

† The pica argument is an old one. Disturbed children, it goes, are more likely to chew paint or lick their fingers after getting them covered with dust (which in cities contains high levels of lead). Therefore, it is argued, it is hardly surprising that the lead burdens of such children are higher than those of normal children who are (it is claimed) less prone to pica. In other words, disturbed children are not disturbed because they have higher lead levels: rather, they have high lead levels because they

with the issue of pica in his study and, although he found an association between the habit and some measures of IQ, he showed convincingly that this was not a relationship which was statistically significant.[39] Yet the Committee failed to mention that finding – despite the fact that Needleman had written three papers (all published before the Committee's report and all easily obtainable) which explained his reasoning.

Not one of those papers was cited, let alone discussed, by the Working Party in its report.[40] Instead the Committee quoted exclusively from Needleman's first published paper – a paper in which Needleman's discussion of pica had been omitted due to lack of space. Needleman was at pains to point out that omission at a symposium, held in London, to which the working party had been invited. None of its 12 members attended. Nonetheless, according to Professor Bryce-Smith and Dr Robert Stephens, 'they were fully briefed by the civil servants who did attend'.[41]

Indeed all the evidence suggests that the working party knew of Needleman's explanation of the pica factor when it wrote its report. Why then, was that explanation ignored? The more so since one of the members of the committee, Professor Michael Rutter, had visited Needleman and concluded, after analysing the data, that pica could be *dismissed* as a cause of the behavioural disorders observed by Needleman – a conclusion Rutter made quite clear in a review of Needleman's work, published in 1980.[42] From the wording of the section in the Lawther report on Needleman's study, it is clear that the committee relied heavily on Rutter's review. Yet it omitted to include Rutter's assessment, namely that the pica factor was not statistically significant. So too, it omitted to mention that Rutter had found that none of the reservations he held about the Needleman study were 'sufficient to invalidate the findings'.[43]

Nor was that the only example of cavalier science on the part of the

---

are disturbed and thus susceptible to pica. As Nick Kollerstrom notes, however, studies have now cast considerable doubt on the pica hypothesis: 'A Scottish study by Moore in 1977 found a clear correlation between mental subnormality and blood lead level measured a few days after birth. It is fairly plain in this instance that the raised lead must have been a cause of the mental subnormality, since this only became apparent years after the measurements had been taken. Clearly pica could not have been responsible.'[38]

committee. The Montreal study, for example, was dismissed because it had cited teachers' reports of disturbed classroom behaviour rather than 'psychometric' tests. 'It will be recalled,' comments Nick Kollerstrom, 'that this survey had taken two groups of children from a school, one classed as "learning disabled" and the other as "normal", and found that the former had five times higher hair lead than the latter. (The Working Party's) criticism is thus surely quite irrelevant.'[44]

In another instance, the Lawther Committee dismissed a series of studies (which had linked high blood lead levels to mental retardation and hyperactivity) on the grounds that they did not take sufficient account of social class variables. Those studies had been conducted by Dr Oliver David of the Downside Medical Centre, Brooklyn, New York. In fact, David was later to tell Bryce-Smith that social factors had been taken into account in all but one of the studies criticised by the committee.[45] The exception was an early study on hyperactivity, published in 1972. That study, David admits, had shown 'a slight (very slight) social class bias'. But the bias was not what one might have expected. 'It was in the wrong direction', says David. 'That is, if there was a difference in social class, it was the hyperactive group not the control group that had more upper-class subjects within it.' All the other studies, it should be noted, showed a lead effect even 'after social class was controlled'.[46]

But whilst the committee was highly critical (frequently, as we have seen, to the point of distortion) of studies which found lead pollution to be a cause of behavioural disorders, it was strangely uncritical of studies which found no such effect. It quoted approvingly a 1974 study by one of its members, Professor Richard Lansdown of the Hospital for Sick Children, Great Ormond Street, London, which had found no differences between the IQ levels and classroom behaviour of children living near a lead smelter and those living further away.[48] That result was hardly surprising, however, for, as Nick Kollerstrom points out: 'It happened that those living furthest from the smelter (and thus having the lower lead levels) were in a different housing area which had a higher proportion of disturbed and delinquent children and a lower average IQ. The comparison of this group with those living near the smelter was used to infer that lead had no effect on IQ or classroom behaviour.'[49] In fact, says Kollerstrom, the 1974

Landsdown survey served as 'a classic "nil result" experiment'. [50]

The publication of the Lawther report, was greeted with dismay bordering on disbelief by environmentalists. For its part, the Conservation Society, in its 'counter-report' *Lead or Health*, commented: 'Concerning the Lawther report, we welcomed its recognition that a problem may exist, but we find its discussion of key aspects so deeply flawed, and its failure to include some of the most important areas of evidence so stultifying as to render it not just largely useless, but its central features dangerously misleading as an assessment of the present state of knowledge.' [51]

Although the Working Party recommended that the lead content of petrol should be 'progressively reduced', it remained committed to the principal shibboleths of the pro-lead lobby. It had 'no doubt', for instance, that a blood-lead level of 35 μg/100 ml provided a firm safety threshold for children. And it was adamant that only 10-20 per cent of inhaled lead is absorbed by the body (other experts suggest 32-69 per cent is a more realistic figure. [52] But its most remarkable conclusion came in paragraph 208 of its report: 'We have seen that in the vast majority of the population, airborne lead, including that derived from petrol, is usually a minor contributor to the body burden. Normally, food is the major source and we have seen no evidence that this is substantially enhanced by contamination by airborne lead.' [53] In effect, the man in the street was being asked to believe that the lead released into the atmosphere from motor cars – accounting for approximately 90 per cent of airborne lead – was somehow disappearing into thin air, harming no-one and accumulating nowhere.

Such an assumption is not only highly implausible, it also flies in the face of the available evidence. A study by Reading's Environmental Health Department, for instance, found that lead levels in the outer leaves of cabbages (those exposed most to lead in the atmosphere) were up to ten times higher than lead levels in the hearts of the cabbages. [54] In Denmark researchers found that atmospheric lead was responsible for 'between 90 and 99 per cent' of the total lead content in the grass grown in rural areas. [55] Nor, apparently, is the contamination restricted to vegetables and grass: sheep, too, have been found to have raised lead-levels as a result of inhaling atmospheric lead or eating grass contaminated by it. [56] Moreover, because lead in 'aerosol' form (that is, as an airborne particle) can be transported for miles before finally coming to rest, the contamination can extend far beyond the original source of pollution. Clair Patterson, a geochemist at the California Institute of Technology, has found that even in the remote Yosemite National Park in the Sierra mountains of California, 'industrial lead brought in as aerosols appears to comprise 50 per cent of lead in soil humus, 90 per cent of lead in sedge plants and 95 per cent of the lead in herbivores and carnivores.'[57] Indeed, Professor Bryce-Smith and Dr Robert Stephens conclude in *Lead or Health*: 'Fall-out of lead is by far the major source of lead in typical food crops consumed by humans and farm animals, even (when) grown in farmland or mountain areas away from main roads and industrial sources.'[58]

In fact, the extent of lead pollution in our food has already reached alarming proportions. As of 1979, the statutory limit for the amount of lead in food was reduced from 2 ppm to 1 ppm: for baby food, the limit was set at 0.2 ppm, in line with WHO standards.[59] At those levels, says Dr Robin Russell Jones, 'there are few places left in the British Isles where (vegetables with a high surface area) can be grown and still considered fit for infant consumption'.[60] Indeed, he points out, food grown within 10 kilometres of Marble Arch is already quite unfit for human consumption – either by infants or adults.[61]

Russell Jones's views are based on a 1975-76 survey, carried out by the Ministry of Agriculture, Fisheries and Food (MAFF), which analysed the lead content of vegetables and herbage on various farms around Britain. Hardly any of the samples taken were found to contain lead levels below the 0.2 ppm standard for baby food.[62] 'In general, crops ranged between 0.2 and 1 ppm in mean lead content,' reports Nick Kollerstrom, 'but a disturbing proportion was above the 1 ppm limit, that is to say it was unfit for consumption by adults.'[63] Levels of lead in 17 samples of potatoes were found to have a mean lead content of 0.7 ppm, whilst 10 samples of barley had a mean lead content of 2.5 ppm.[64] One farm, downwind from an industrial site, had such high lead levels that, in the opinion of Kollerstrom, it was 'contaminated to a degree where it is probably unsuitable for any food production'. Meanwhile, in 1980, the Nottingham Environment Advisory Council reported that blackberries picked from hedgerows and banks along the A52 contained lead levels in excess of 6 ppm –

and that jam prepared from the fruit 'contained 20 times the legal maximum for infant food'. [66]

Such figures are an appalling indictment of the extent to which we are contaminating our environment. Indeed, it is now estimated that most foods crops in Britain now have lead levels 100 times higher than those found in pre-industrial times. [67] For its part, however, MAFF has tried to play down the problem. When, for instance, Nick Kollerstrom made further inquiries about the 1979 MAFF survey and the high levels of lead it reported in food crops, he was told that the contamination was due to the land being treated with sewage sludge (which contains in the region of 400 ppm of lead.) [68] Yet, says Kollerstrom, 'the report makes quite clear which crops came from sludge-treated land and which not'. [69] Moreover, those samples were not (as a MAFF official suggested) taken from experimental plots especially treated with contaminated sludge. [70] In another instance, when Kollerstrom asked about the extent of lead contamination in barley, he was sent a list of lead levels in wheat. [71] Those levels averaged 0.1 ppm of lead. MAFF officials went on to claim that 'their unpublished data is all below 0.2 ppm,' – in which case, comments Kollerstrom, 'it is up to them to explain why their most recent published data is almost all above it.' [72]

As a last resort, MAFF tried to explain away the results of its 1979 survey by arguing that they were the consequence of faulty procedures and poor analytical techniques. Thus, Kollerstrom was told: 'Most of the participating laboratories used a method which could not accurately quantify levels of lead below 2-3 mg/kg in dry matter.' [73] Since 2-3 mg/kg is the equivalent of 2-3 ppm, that statement hardly provides grounds for reassurance. Indeed, as Kollerstrom remarks: 'If all measurements made below 2 or 3 ppm were unreliable, then this would show a strange degree of incompetence in an HMSO publication giving the most recent data on Britain's most important pollutant. Do their competent measurements only begin at a level 3 times higher than the statutory health limit?' [74] Or is it that the Ministry would rather not admit that our children are being systematically poisoned?

If environmentalists were dismayed by the Lawther report, the government was delighted. Here, after all, was a team of experts –

described as the 'most formidable' ever to 'scrutinise the issue'[75] – which was telling the country that there was no cause for alarm over leaded petrol. One can imagine the consternation when rumours began to circulate around Whitehall in early 1981 that two members of the working party had found positive evidence that lead was indeed harmful to childrens' health. The two members were Dr William Yule, of the Institute of Psychiatry at London University, and Dr Richard Lansdown. Throughout 1980, the year in which the Lawther Committee was collecting evidence and writing its report, Yule and Lansdown had been analysing the IQ levels and school performance of a group of children in Greenwich.[76] That study found that 'children with the lowest blood lead levels scored consistently better on tests of reading, spelling and intelligence' than those with higher blood lead levels.[77] Moreover, that effect was noted at blood lead levels above 13 μg/100 ml, one IQ point being knocked off for every μg/100 ml of lead above that level.[78] Indeed, after such factors as social class and age had been taken into account, Yule and Lansdown found a 7 point IQ deficit in the high lead group.[79] Responding to criticisms of the study in a letter to *The Times*, Yule wrote: 'We concluded that there remained a small but real relationship between blood lead level and children's attainment . . . the scientific evidence at present *does* support the view that there is a connection between blood lead levels and school performance.'[80]

Although the Yule and Lansdown study was not published until September 1981 (the authors had great difficulty in finding a journal which would accept their paper: the *British Medical Journal*, whose pro-lead editorial stance was notorious at the time, rejected it on the grounds that its statistics were faulty) a draft copy was circulated around the DHSS early in 1981.[81] At the same time, Ministers were confronted with a letter, written by Sir Henry Yellowlees, Chief Medical Officer of the Department of Health. The letter had been written to the Permanent Secretary at the Department of Education and Science and it took a very different line to that of the Lawther committee. After discussing the findings of *Lead and Health*, Sir Henry wrote:

'I must now make my own position clear. A year ago when the Lawther report was published there was a degree of uncertainty, but since then further evidence has accrued which, though not itself wholly conclusive, nevertheless supports the view that:

a) Even at low blood levels there is a negative correlation between blood lead levels and IQ of which the simplest explanation is that the lead produces these effects:

b) Lead in petrol is a major contributor to blood lead acting through the food chain as well as by inhalation.

Further research is being mounted but we are dealing here with the biological sciences where truly conclusive evidence may be unobtainable and it is therefore doubtful whether there is anything to be gained by deferring a decision until the results of further research become available.

There is a strong likelihood that lead in petrol is permanently reducing the IQ of many of our children. Although the reduction amounts to only a few percentage points, some hundreds of thousands of children are affected and as Chief Medical Officer I have advised my Secretary of State that action should be taken now to reduce markedly the lead content of petrol in use in the United Kingdom.

The risk to children is now shown to be too great for me to take any other course and I am therefore conveying this advice to you as Permanent Secretary in DES and I am copying the letter to the Permanent Secretaries at the Home Office and the Department of the Environment being the other Government departments to which I owe responsibility.

You will know that several other major industrial nations faced with similar problems have opted for lead-free petrol or for petrol with a very low lead level despite the substantial costs and the energy penalties so incurred.

I regard this as a very serious issue on which I should give you my opinion as Chief Medical Officer.'[82]

Serious it was indeed, and there is little doubt that, together with the Yules and Lansdown report, Yellowlees's letter forced the government's hand and compelled it to act. Thus, eventually in May 1981, the government announced that the lead content of petrol was to be reduced by 1986 from 0.4 grams/litre to 0.15 grams/litre. The government refused, however, to go for a complete ban on petrol. Nonetheless, it was clear that the establishment's ivory tower was beginning to crumble.

Although environmentalists welcomed the new limits, there was bitter disappointment that the government had stopped so far short of a complete ban on leaded petrol. Even at the new level of 0.15 grams/litre, it was pointed out, some 3,000 tons of lead would still be pumped into Britain's air every year.[83] The time had clearly come for a concerted campaign to push for lead-free petrol and, in January 1982, the Campaign for Lead-Free Air (CLEAR) was born. CLEAR's director was the veteran campaigner and journalist, Des Wilson, best known for his work at SHELTER on behalf of the homeless. Immediately after it was launched at a press conference in London, CLEAR went into the attack, leaking the Yellowlees letter to *The Times*.[84]

That leak was followed by an international symposium organised by CLEAR held in May 1982. The chairman of the symposium was Professor Michael Rutter, a former member of the Lawther Committee who, it will be remembered, had reviewed Needleman's work for the working party. In his summing up, he made it clear that he had abandoned many of the views he had held earlier, not least the suggestion that lead in petrol contributes only 10 per cent to the body's lead burden. That figure, he said, was inaccurate – the real figure was closer to 30 per cent.[85] 'On the hypothesis that low level lead exposure leads to psychological impairment,' he told the symposium, 'the implication is that it would be safer in practice and scientifically more appropriate to act as if the hypothesis was true, rather than to continue to act as if it was not true.'

'The risk', he went on, 'seems to be substantially more than a trivial one, at least in some individuals, since the effects are likely to be of practical importance in causing impairment of functioning. The implication is that we now know enough to warrant taking such public health actions as are likely to reduce lead pollution in the environment, provided such actions do not have other hazards and provided that they are not prohibitively expensive. The removal of lead would seem to be one of those worthwhile and safe public health actions. The evidence suggests that the removal of lead from petrol would have quite a substantial effect on reducing lead pollution and the costs are quite modest by any reasonable standard . . . In my view, the reduction of lead in the environment should make some worthwhile differences to some children and that ought to constitute a quite sufficient justification for action now.'[86]

The response of the government was perhaps predictable. It continued to quote the Lawther report for all it was worth – a strange response given that so much doubt had been voiced about its conclusions.

Whilst in Britain environmentalists were campaigning to *cut* the lead content of petrol, in America they were battling against attempts by industry to *raise* permitted lead levels. The ensuing battle (both between environmentalists and the oil refining industry, and within the Environmental Protection Agency) throws a none too flattering light on the process by which environmental standards are set in the US – and, by implication, elsewhere. Although the US Clean Air Act Amendment of 1977 had set a strict limit on the amount of lead allowed in petrol, it had given small refineries leave to add lead to petrol at the old levels until their equipment was replaced. The result, as Eliot Marshall reports in *Science*, was that 'some astute entrepreneurs saw the opportunity . . . and set themselves up as "small refiners" – actually blenders – in the high-lead gasoline business. They have done well, buying poor quality gasoline, mixing it with relatively large amounts of lead, and marketing it well below the price set by other domestic refiners.'[87]

Moreover, when the decision to phase out leaded petrol had originally been taken, the EPA had allowed refineries to 'average out' the levels of leaded and unleaded petrol so that, in total, the lead content did not exceed 0.5 grams/US gallon. Inevitably, perhaps, as the refineries produced more unleaded petrol, so they added more lead to their leaded petrol – the *average* lead content still being kept within the limits.[88]

To combat those anomalies and loopholes, the EPA proposed new regulations which would have set a limit of 1.1 grams/US gallon of lead in petrol, excusing only the smallest refineries from abiding by the new laws.[89]

EPA officials had reckoned, however, without the influence of their director, Anna Gorsuch, a Reagan appointee who has done more than anyone to 'rape' the EPA. In April 1982, at a meeting with lobbyists for the lead industry, she is reported to have said that she hoped 'to drastically revise or abolish' the lead standards. More interesting was her behaviour towards representatives of a small refinery. As Eliot Marshall reports: 'The best documented of the refiner meetings took place at 10.00 a.m. on December 11th 1981, and included Gorsuch, Larry Morgan of Senator Schmitt's staff, two other EPA officials, Gerald Preston, then Vice-President of Thriftway Gasoline Company of New Mexico, and two consulting attorneys for Thriftway, William Cockrell and Edward Shipper. The meeting arranged by Senator Schmitt (the refinery was in his constituency of New Mexico) was intended to give Thriftway a chance to ask Gorsuch for a special waiver allowing the company to add more lead to its gasoline. Gorsuch did not grant the waiver in writing. But, according to four participants in the meeting, she gave her word that she would not enforce the existing standards, and she encouraged Thriftway to ignore them.'[90]

That evidence came out in a 1982 hearing held by the US House of Representatives. At the hearing, it was learnt from a subpoenaed document, written by Shipper, that: 'Gorsuch noted that EPA's lead phase-down regulations would probably be revised and perhaps even abolished during the course of the upcoming rulemaking, in accordance with Vice President Bush's expressed intentions . . . We all thanked her and then left to meet John Hernandez for a social visit. Larry Morgan, however, remained behind with Gorsuch momentarily. When he came out he told us that the administrator explained to him that she couldn't actually tell us to go out and break the law, but she hoped that we had gotten the message.'[91]

In the event, however, EPA officials did not bow to pressure from Gorsuch, or indeed from Vice President Bush. In September 1982, the new regulations went through. The EPA estimates that they will reduce airborne lead concentrations by 31 per cent.[92]

In Britain, the debate over lead levels still rages. The main objection, posed by government and industry alike, is that going 'lead-free' would cost the country dear in both financial terms and in terms of spiralling fuel bills. Although evidence from those countries which have started to phase out leaded petrol suggests the contrary, the government has stuck to its guns: lead-free petrol is an unnecessary expense. But is it? Particularly when set against the enormous financial burden of caring for the thousands of children we are poisoning each year. And, surely, it would be preferable to pay the price now rather than pick up the bill in thirty to forty years time after we have witnessed a tragedy on a scale far greater than that of either asbestos or thalidomide? Quite simply, which should the government be putting first: the future of our children? Or the profits of our oil companies?

Perhaps the last word should go to those who have done most to expose the lead scandal in Britain, Professor Bryce-Smith and Robert Stephens on the Conservation Society's Pollution Working Party. For although, since they wrote *Lead or Health?*, the government has reduced the lead content of petrol and now recommends that children with blood-lead levels above 25 μg/100 ml should be treated by a doctor, their remarks still stand.[93] They write:

'The technically unnecessary but still convenient adulteration of petrol by lead has grown to the dimensions of a crime against the human race, no less: a casual crime committed in the blinkered pursuit of business profits, cynically concealed and perpetuated by political influence and the cosmetic arts of public relations, and the insidious cause of untold loss, suffering and social disadvantage among people who mostly have no idea what is happening.'

Leaded petrol is a crime. Should it really go unpunished?

POSTSCRIPT

After the war, the industrial world witnessed a revolution so quiet in its coming and so insidious in its effects that it was not until the late sixties that the majority of us woke up to its consequences. That revolution was born in the marriage of science and technology: industry exploited it – and the environment suffered from its ravages. Whereas the scientists of the past were often viewed with suspicion, if not downright hostility, the new breed of post-war scientists were adulated. A few years at university, peering down microscopes and making notes (albeit meticulous notes) and the science graduate was expected to understand the world. More than that, he was expected to change it: set apart from the rest of us by his learning and his jargon, his was the task of leading us into the brave new world of science fiction.

Such was the respect accorded to science that, in 1966, Vice President Hubert Humphrey told an audience of young scientists: 'For the year 2000, we can see some really far-out developments: the virtual elimination of bacterial and viral diseases; the correction of hereditary defects through the modification of genetic chemistry; the stepping up of our food supply through the use of large scale ocean farming and the fabrication of synthetic proteins. In space, the landing of men on Mars and the establishment of a permanent unmanned research station on that planet and the creation in the laboratory of artificial life. This can indeed be the Age of Miracles. It will be your age.'

Few now expect such developments – even if they were actually desirable – to take place. Even those that Humphrey predicted would be commonplace by the 1980s now seem pipedreams: witness his belief that by 1986 we would have a permanent base on the moon. But, I would contend, it is precisely that euphoric, awe-inspired reverence which Humphrey – and indeed most of us – showed towards science which was (and still is) the root cause of many of the cover-ups I have described. Scientists are as human as the industrialists who control their laboratories – as susceptible to bribes, corruption and sheer power-seeking as the rest of us.

Like us, they are ruled by everyday concerns (the mortgage, the need to provide for a family, the fear of failure or criticism) and like us, they must ultimately succumb to the pressure of market forces – whether or not those forces are controlled by capitalism or communism. Just as successive governments have been prepared to water down environmental legislation, fudge safety levels for exposure to chemicals, and underplay dangers in order to save industry from bankruptcy, so scientists are prepared to cut corners and believe 'the best' for the sake of their companies and their careers. The problem is that we believe them despite the fact that expertise is as saleable a commodity as gold: and despite our all too cynical knowledge that 'he who pays the piper calls the tune'.

Of course, there are those who are prepared to exploit a drug or a chemical – even if it has been proven to be dangerous to human health or the environment – for the sake of profit, power or personal prestige. One is reminded instantly of those companies who continue to export drugs and chemicals banned in the West to Third World countries – and one is reminded too of President Reagan's decision to rescind curbs on such exports. But for the most part the motive for cover-up or downright political chicanery is less sinister: unprepared to rock the boat, politicians, industrialists and scientists alike are psychologically unable to see that they might be wrong.

Perhaps that should not surprise us – particularly where the scientists are concerned. The motives of businessmen and politicians are easy to define: profit and prestige. But what are we to make of the motives of scientists? On the one hand one has the single-mindedness of a Robert Oppenheimer, so preoccupied with his project that he was unable to see its consequences until too late. And yet, after his 'baby' – the first atomic bomb – had been exploded, he was to write: 'We knew the world would not be the same. A few people laughed, a few people cried. Most people were silent. I remembered the line from the

Hindu scripture, the *Bhagavad Gita*: Vishnu is trying to persuade the Prince that he should do his duty and to impress him takes on his multi-armed form and says "Now I am become death, destroyer of worlds". I suppose we all thought that one way or another.'[1]

On the other hand, one has the run-of-the-mill scientist whose main motive is to earn his living. Of these, Hank Schumacher, one of America's top weapon designers, has commented: 'Once they're in it (military research) very few people think much about it. My colleagues who work on nuclear devices don't do it for a reason. They do it because they are nuclear physicists.'[2]

Cocooned in their everyday world, both scientists and industrialists often tend to see critics as 'troublemakers', the 'vocal minority' out to destroy society and all that goes with it. Take, for example, a speech given by Werner Gebauer, President of the International Group of National Associations of Agrochemical Manufacturers, at a conference held in September 1981 in Zurich: 'Even if the claims of the environment fanatics are scientifically untenable and often cause the people actually involved in the industry and agriculture merely to shake their heads, the ecology movement, with the help of the media – for whom agrochemicals have become a perennial and profitable topic – has still managed to create a good deal of uncertainty and suspicion among broad sectors of the public.'[3]

Or again, take the memorandum leaked to US Friends of the Earth from the Secretary of the US Department of the Interior, Andrew Bailey, to the environmental department of his office: 'Inflammatory words such as disturbed, devastated, defiled, ravaged, gouged, scarred, and destroyed should not be used (in environmental impact statements). These are words used by the Sierra Club, Friends of the Earth, environmentalists, homosexuals, ecologists and other ideological eunuchs opposed to developing mineral resources.'[4]

In such an atmosphere, it is scarcely surprising that a fortress mentality develops. Indeed, once overcome by it, there is a strong tendency for companies and large institutions to become 'States within States', with one department vying with another in an attempt to ensure their own self-preservation and self-aggrandisement. Nowhere in this more so than in the nuclear industry. As Duncan Burns, the foremost historian of Britain's nuclear industry, points out: 'Authorities and boards become vested interests, eager for more power, for larger staffs and large empires, anxious to conceal or explain away what has gone wrong.'[5, 6]

Inevitably, that fortress mentality becomes a hothouse for cover-ups. Once a decision has been made – particularly if millions of pounds or dollars have gone into making it – it is difficult for any company or institution to go back on it without losing face. It is equally difficult for those involved in making a decision not to develop a psychological stake in seeing it implemented. Ally that reluctance to reconsider decisions or to tolerate criticism with the incredible power enjoyed by the majority of large institutions and one has the perfect recipe for dangerously wrong-headed thinking.

The more so when there are vast sums of money involved, and when critics are seen as the enemy. After all it takes a great deal of courage for a junior executive to tell his seniors that a new product they are about to market after years of research is a health hazard. Far easier to hide behind the comforting, uncommitted language of a scientific report and reassure oneself that the phrase 'there is no evidence' really does mean an outright denial of danger – rather than a meek admission that no one really knows for certain.

But whilst it is easy to understand how a cover-up begins, it is more than difficult to know how to stop it – or still worse prevent it from happening. The problem lies in that marriage between science, technology and industry which I mentioned at the beginning of this chapter. For, so long as the health of industry is seen as more important than the health of the general public, the cover-up society is ensured. Nothing short of a radical change in our values will prevent it.

Time is of the essence. Wedded to an economic system which, as one commentator puts it, 'values American cats over West African people because the former can pay for their food while the latter frequently cannot', we are rapidly destroying the very basis of our survival on earth. The predictions are frightening: one-third of the world's ice-free land area is expected to be converted to desert through overgrazing and deforestation by the end of the century (already an area equivalent of twice the size of Belgium is lost to desertification every year); half of the world's tropical rainforests will probably be lost within a hundred years (assuming that the rate of their destruction remains at the present staggering twenty-five acres a minute) and then there is the certainty of climatic change as a result of deforestation and the destruction of other vegetable cover.

To be sure there will be those 'experts' who tell us all is well and that there is nothing to worry about. But if there is one message in COVER-UP it is that the public should not trust the *ex cathedra* statements of professional scientists. I hope, too, that another message is clear: for every cover-up perpetrated through greed, there is another perpetrated through complacency. It may be comforting to take refuge in conspiracy theories, but that misses the point. If there is a conspiracy, we are all part of it. It is we who demand the goods from industry: who demand that they are cheap and who do not question how they are manufactured often until it is too late. And if to maintain our standard of living, industry has resorted to devious and deceitful methods – and got away with it – unquestioning consumerism is a willing accomplice. Given resolve it is a battle we can win. But not until we break the economic and political marriage between science and the state. That, perhaps, is the real lesson of the 'cover-up'.

SOURCE NOTES

Introduction
1. 'The Medical/Industrial Complex.' *Lancet* 2, (1973).
2. Subcommittee on Crime of the House Judiciary Committee US House of Representatives, 1980. Testimony of George Miller.

Chapter 1: The Death of Karen Silkwood

1. J. Barton, *Intensified Nuclear Safeguards and Civil Liberties*, Nuclear Regulatory Commission, Washington D.C., 1975 (Contract No. AT 49-24 0190).
2. J. Barton, *op.cit.* 1975, p.27. Although Barton does not deal specifically with the methods of interrogation which might be used, he warns: ' . . . detention could be used as a step in a very troubling interrogation scheme – perhaps employing lie detectors or even torture. The normal deterrent to such practices – inadmissibility of evidence in court – would be ineffective under the conditions of a nuclear emergency.'
3. Howard Kohn, 'Nuclear Power on Trial', *Rolling Stone,* 4.5.78, p.48.
4. J. Garrison, 'The Mysterious Case of Karen Silkwood', *The Ecologist,* Vol. 9 Nos. 8/9, Nov/Dec 1979, p.294.
5. Excellent accounts of Silkwood's childhood and background appear in: Howard Kohn, 'Malignant Giant', *Rolling Stone*, 27.3.75; and Richard Rashke, *Karen Silkwood: Union Sister*, Oil, Chemical and Atomic Workers' Union/National Organisation of Women, Washington D.C., 1979.
6. K. Tucker and E. Walters, *Plutonium and the Workplace; An Assessment of Health and Safety Procedures for Workers at the Kerr-McGee FFTF Plutonium Fuel Fabrication Facility*, Environmental Policy Institute, Washington D.C., 1979.
7. K.Z. Morgan, Testimony before the Subcommittee on Energy and the Environment of the Committee on Small Businesses; *Problems in the Accounting for and Safeguarding of Special Nuclear Materials*, US House of Representatives (94th Congress, 2nd Session) Washington D.C., 1976, pp.3-4.
8. S. Nelson and K. Tucker, Statement before Subcommittee on Energy and the Environment of the Committee on Small Businesses; *Problems in the Accounting for and Safeguarding of Special Nuclear Materials*, US

House of Representatives (94th Congress, 2nd Session), Washington D.C., 1976, pp.230-231: See also, K. Tucker and E. Walters, *op.cit.* 1979, pp.23, 70-72.

9. J. Smith, Sworn Deposition, US District Court for the Western District of Oklahoma, 1978.

10. K. Tucker and E. Walters, *op.cit.* 1979, p.52.

11. *Panorama*, The Case of Karen Silkwood, BBC, 1979.

12. J. Smith, Sworn Deposition, *op.cit.* 1978: K. Tucker and E. Walters, *op.cit.* 1979, p.33; R. Rashke, *op.cit.* 1978, p.3.

13. Howard Kohn, 'Malignant Giant', *Rolling Stone*, 27.3.75 (Offprint), p.3.

14. K. Tucker and E. Walters, *op.cit.* 1979, pp.50-51: R. Rashke, *op.cit.* 1978, p.3: H. Kohn, *op.cit.* 1975 (Offprint) p.3.

15. R. Rashke, *op.cit.* 1978, p.10.

16. R. Rashke, *op.cit.* 1978, p.10: K. Tucker and E. Walters, *op.cit.* 1979, p.62: D. Sheehan, 'Affidavit supporting Brief in Opposition to quash the Subpoenas Duces issued to witnesses Althowe, Wormelli, Benson and Leyrer,' US District Court for the Western District of Oklahoma, 1978, p.6.

17. AEC investigators in 1973 found that one laboratory analyst, William S. Dotter, had indeed been touching up negatives. Dotter, however, claimed that he had only touched up defects in the film itself, not evidence of defects in the fuel rods. The AEC accepted that explanation. (See: Deborah Shapley, 'Breeder Reactors: Fast Flux Fuel Rods subject of Silkwood Charges', *Science*, Vol. 199, 3.3.78, pp.956-958.)

18. Mazzochi, Testimony before US District Court for the Western District of Oklahoma, quoted in *The Nashville Tennessean*, 1.4.79.

19. Telephone conversation taped by Steve Wodka of OCAW, 1974.

20. R. Rashke, *op.cit.* 1978, p.4: H. Kohn, *op.cit.* 1975 (Offprint) p.3.

21. Interview with Daniel Sheehan, Washington D.C., 1980.

22. J. Garrison, *op.cit.* 1979, p.293: H. Kohn, *op.cit.* 1975 (Offprint) p.4: R. Rashke, *op.cit.* 1978, p.5.

23. H. Kohn, *op.cit.* 1975, p.4.

24. J. Gofman, Testimony before US District Court of the Western District of Oklahoma, 1978, pp.36-44.

25. R. Rashke, *op.cit.* 1978, p.5.

26. D. Sheehan: Affidavit Brief in Opposition to Quash the Subpoenas Duces issued to witnesses Althowe, Wormelli, Benson and Leyrer, US District Court for the Western District of Oklahoma, 1978, p.9: J. Garrison, *op.cit.* 1979, p.293.

27. R. Rashke, *op.cit.* 1978, p.5.

28. Ibid. p.5.

29. J. Garrison, *op.cit.* 1979, p.294: D. Sheehan, *op.cit.* 1978, p.10. According to Rashke (*op.cit.* 1978, p.5.): 'Karen's landlord later told Silkwood investigators there was a trap door in the ceiling of her bedroom

closet that the K.M. inspectors apparently didn't find during the first day of the search.'

30. R. Rashke, *op.cit.* 1978, p.7: D. Sheehan, *op.cit.* 1978, p.12. The reason given for allowing the K.M. men access to Karen's car was so they could check it for contamination. This was in fact done.

31. D. Sheehan, *op.cit.* 1978, pp.11-12.

32. R. Rashke, *op.cit.* 1978, p.7.

33. Ibid. p.7.

34. A.O. Pipkin, 'Accident Reconstruction Laboratory Report', Dallas, Texas, 1974.

35. H. Kohn, 'The Case of Karen Silkwood', *Rolling Stone*, 13.1.77, p.32: R. Rashke, *op.cit.* 1978, pp.7-9.

36. J. Garrison, *op.cit.* 1979, p.295.

37. H. Kohn, *op.cit.* 13.1.77, p.31.

38. *Panorama, op.cit.* 1979: R. Rashke, *op.cit.* p.5. The plutonium that contaminated Karen Silkwood came from pellet lot number 29. She never had access to it.

39. H. Kohn, *op.cit.* 13.1.77, p.31.

40. H. Kohn, 'Karen Silkwood was Right in Plutonium Scandal', *Rolling Stone*, 20.10.77.

41. H. Kohn, *op.cit.* 13.1.77, p.31.

42. Ibid. p.34.

43. K. Tucker, 'Karen Silkwood Union Organiser', NOW, Washington D.C., 1975, p.34.

44. Interview with D. Sheehan, Washington D.C., 1980.

45. H. Kohn, *op.cit.* 13.1.77, p.36.

46. Interview with D. Sheehan, Washington, D.C., 1980. Also, D. Sheehan, *op.cit.* 1978, p.16.

47. J. Garrison, *op.cit.* 1979, p.296.

48. H. Kohn, *op.cit.* 13.1.77, p.38. According to Kohn, Stockton recognised the voice of the caller as that of Lawrence Olson.

49. J. Srouji, Testimony before Subcommittee on Energy and the Environment of the Committee on Small Businesses; *Problems in the Accounting for and Safeguarding of Special Nuclear Materials*, US House of Representatives (94th Congress, 2nd Session) Washington D.C., 1976, p.247.

50. D. Sheehan, *op.cit.* 1978, p.18.

51. The Karen Silkwood Public Education Fund, *The Silkwood Case; A Battle for Civil Liberties*, Washington D.C., 1976. D. Sheehan, *op.cit.* 1978, p.19 ff. See also J. Seigenthaler, Testimony before Subcommittee on Energy and the Environment of the Committee on Small Businesses, *Problems in the Accounting for and Safeguarding of Special Nuclear Materials*, US House of Representatives (94th Congress, 2nd Session) Washington D.C., 1976, p.315 ff.

52. H. Kohn, *op.cit.* 13.1.77, p.37: D. Sheehan, *op.cit.* 1978, p.20.

53. Interview with D. Sheehan, Washington D.C., 1980.

54. Ibid.

55. D. Sheehan, *op.cit.* 1978, p.28.

56. D. Sheehan, *op.cit.* 1978, p.32: Interview with D. Sheehan, Washington D.C., 1980.

57. George O'Toole, 'America's Secret Police Network', *Penthouse*, December 1976, p.79.

58. Ibid. p.202.

59. Interview with D. Sheehan, Washington D.C., 1980.

60. Interview with D. Sheehan, Washington D.C., 1980. See also local Oklahoma newspaper reports for July and August 1961; and Deposition of J. Seigenthaler before Edna L. Gardner, Notary, 16.12.77. Seigenthaler was Assistant to the Attorney General, Robert P. Kennedy, at the time of Bohanan's appointment.

61. 'Ghostly Case: Silkwood Trail', *San Francisco Examiner*, 4.3.79, p.1. and p.10 (Section A).

Chapter 2: Down in the Dumps

1. *Report of the Royal Commission on Environmental Pollution*, HMSO, London, 1978, p.113. The figures quoted are for 1971.

2. A. Pickaver, *The Pollution of the North Sea*, Greenpeace publications, London, 1981. The exact figure for the total amount of waste being dumped into these seas by Britain (and indeed other countries) is difficult to determine. The figure of 23.5 million tonnes for Britain is drawn from the 8th meeting of the Standing Advisory Committee for Scientific Advice, Oslo Convention, 1980. The House of Lords Select Committee on Science and Technology in its 1981 report, *Hazardous Waste Disposal*, gives a figure of 45.21 tonnes dumped in all by Britain at sea. The Select Committee also gives different figures to Greenpeace on the amount of industrial waste disposed by Britain at sea: 0.60 million tons as opposed to 2.9 million tons, (see Pickaver, *op.cit.* 1981, p.13: House of Lords Select Committee on Science and Technology, *Hazardous Waste Disposal*, HMSO, London, 1981, p.10).

3. A. Pickaver (*op.cit.* 1981) gives a very different picture of pollution in the North Sea – defined to include the English Channel, the Skaggerak and Kattegat, the Irish Sea but not the Baltic – to that presented by the British Government. According to Pickaver (p.9) 'the wastes being dumped into the North Sea are potentially the greatest threat to the survival of life in the water'. Altogether in 1979 (the last year at the time of writing for which figures are available) some 79.4 million tonnes of waste – 8.8 million tonnes of industrial waste, 8.8 million tonnes of sewage sludge and 61.8 million tonnes of dredgings – were 'registered as being directly dumped in the North Sea'. Almost one third of the industrial waste and 96 per cent of the sewage sludge was dumped by Britain (Pickaver, *op.cit.* 1981, pp.13-14: Brian Price, 'The Manchester Goldfish Pond', *Guardian*, 22.10.81).

Among the industrial wastes being dumped were PCBs (insulators used in the production of neon lights and other electrical equipment); the pesticides DDT, Dieldrin and Aldrin (all banned in the US); and heavy metals such as mercury, zinc and cadmium. Pickaver also gives evidence of industrial wastes being dumped illegally.

Legal and illegal, the wastes are already causing severe ecological degradation. PCBs dumped in the River Rhine are 'directly leading to the extinction of the native common seal population in the Wadden Islands' (p.12). Between 20 and 50 per cent of the fish caught in the German Bight are deemed unfit for human consumption, the contamination now being linked to the dumping of wastes containing titanium. Of the total tonnage of industrial wastes dumped in the North Sea, almost 15 per cent is acknowledged to be potentially carcinogenic (B. Price, *op.cit.* 22.10.81).

Pickaver foresees industry and government alike continuing to use the North Sea as Europe's most convenient dustbin well into the 1980s. Moreover the clear trend (judged by the tonnage of wastes being authorised for dumping) is towards an increase in the amount of industrial waste – by far the most toxic – being dumped. Thus, despite a significant drop in the tonnage of dredgings authorised for dumping in 1980 (19.2 million tonnes down on 1979) the amount of industrial waste authorised was 600,000 tonnes up on 1979, whilst the amount of sewage sludge was up by 6.2 million tonnes (pp.13-15, Tables 1-5). Whether or not authorised tonnage is exceeded in practice will not be known until the official figures are published.

To date, Britain has resisted international efforts to tighten restrictions on dumping in the North Sea – her principal defence being that territorial waters have stronger current and carry the pollutants away (p.16). 90 per cent of the permits granted for dumping industrial wastes in 1980 were issued to Britain (p.15, Table 5). In evidence to the 1981 House of Lords Select Committee on *Hazardous Waste Disposal* (*op.cit.* 1981, p.11), experts from the Government's Environmental Safety Group at Harwell claimed that international conventions on sea dumping were 'overprotective' and that they did not 'consider the total environment'. It could be argued, they said, that 'sea disposal of waste materials is a technique by which man speeds up the materials' return to the ocean . . . '

4. M. Waldichuck, 'Review of the Problems in The Assessment of Sublethal Effects of Pollutants in the Sea' *Philosophical Transactions of the Royal Society* (*Biological Services*), vol.286, London, 1979.

5. According to an investigation carried out by the Ministry of Agriculture, Fisheries and Food in 1982, Britain is responsible for 'dumping 90 per cent of all the man-made radioactive wastes entering the world's oceans'. The MAFF investigation endorsed previous criticisms (notably by the Royal Commission on Environmental Pollution) of Britain's programme for monitoring radioactive wastes. The Royal Commission had described the programme on 'the minimum consistent with public and scientific

credibility'. The MAFF investigation agreed and warned that even that minimum programme was in danger of breaking down. 'See: Richard Norton-Taylor, 'Nuclear Checks "Near Collapse" ', *Guardian* 14.6.82.

6. P. Bunyard, 'Nuclear Power – The Grand Illusion', *The Ecologist*, Vol.10. No.4 May 1980, p.125. See also Pickaver, *op.cit*, pp.10-11. Pickaver gives a higher figure (150,000 curies) for the amount of caesium released annually from Windscale. He reports that, between 1972 and 1976, Windscale and its French counterpart Cap de La Hague 'released, respectively, 902,000 and 102,000 curies of radioactivity' including isotopes of strontium, plutonium and caesium. As a direct result of reprocessing at Windscale, 'one quarter to one half tonne of plutonium now lies in the Irish Sea'.

7. A. Tucker, 'Radioactivity Levels Point to Dumping', *Guardian,* 1979. A. Pickaver (*op.cit.* 1981, p.11) also points out: 'On the coast of North-East Russia, radioactive pollution directly attributable to Windscale has been shown to be six times that accountable to radioactive fallout from the atmospheric tests of the fifties and sixties.'

8. Of particular concern is the build-up of plutonium-241 off the Cumbrian coast – the direct result of reprocessing at Windscale. Because it is a beta-emitter, plutonium-241 was assumed to pose a fairly low biological hazard (unlike plutonium-239) and there are no official controls placed on its discharge – although British Nuclear Fuels cut the amount discharged from 40,000 curies in 1970 to 20,000 curies in 1980. Official controls are expected to be introduced in 1983.

By 1980, 381,527 curies of plutonium-241 had built up in the sediment off Windscale – and contrary to expectations, they had not been dispersed by local currents. 'That is potentially serious in its own right for, quite apart from contamination of food chains, sediments move shoreward, materials can easily be resuspended as particles in the atmosphere', says Anthony Tucker of *Guardian*. 'But there is a worse aspect of the problem. Plutonium-241 decays to Americium-241 which has a half-life of 433 years and which, in turn, decays Neptunium-237 which has a half-life of around 2 million years. Both of these isotopes are alpha-emitters. That is to say they are among the most biologically hazardous of materials . . . virtually nothing is known about (the) specific effects of (Americium-241) in humans.' See: A. Tucker, 'Something that will not go away', *The Guardian*, 16.7.81.

9. 'Cadmium in Shellfish', *The Times*, 9.6.76. See also M. Holdgate *et.al. The World Environment 1972-1982*. UNEP/Tycooly International Publishing Ltd., Dublin 1982, p.94: 'Metal concentrations generally are known to have risen in oysters on the Connecticut coast of the United States by 50 per cent to 100 per cent between 1933-35 and the 1970s . . . ' Erik Eckholm (*Down to Earth*, Pluto, London, 1982, p.81) reports: 'In the late 1970s, 26 per cent of the shellfish grounds off thirteen US States were

closed to commercial harvesting because of unsafe contamination'.

10. A. Tucker, 'Toxic Logic – the Cadmium Poisoning Threat', *Guardian*, 22.1.79.

11. 'Will they save the Mediterranean?' *Ambio* (Special Report), Vol. VI, No. 6, 1977. Also: *The Polluted Seas*, Earthscan Press Briefing Document, No. 7, Earthscan, London, 1977.

12. A. Tucker, *The Toxic Metals*, Pan/Ballantine Books, London, 1972, pp.15-87. Reino Watanuki, 'Mercury and Kepone: Two Killers on Two Continents', *Alternatives*, Winter, 1978, pp.4-23. There is still considerable controversy over when the first cases of 'Minemata disease' began to appear: some date the disaster from 1953, others from 1956.

13. A. Tucker, *op.cit.* 1972, pp.15-16. December 1953 saw the first human to fall victim to the disease. In 1954, 12 cases were diagnosed, 5 died; 15 cases were diagnosed in 1955, 3 died; and in 1956, there were 50 cases of whom 10 died.

14. A. Tucker, *op.cit.* 1972, p.15. The figures for those killed or disabled by Minemata disease are the subject of much debate. Tucker's figure of 43 dead and 68 permanently disabled is drawn from *Minemata Disease* (Kumanoto University, Japan, 1968). Tucker cautions, however, that: 'The nature of the poisoning involved, organic mercury, is such that these numbers represent only the obvious tip of a much wider and more sinister pyramid of damage' (p.15). He points out that in Minemata only those with *advanced* symptoms of the disease were recorded as victims: 'The official figures, whether deliberately or not, therefore *minimise* the scale of poisoning' (p.29). Tucker estimates that some 5,000 people – 'more than half of the exposed population' – may have been affected, the degree of damage suffered varying according to such factors as age (p.30). Elsewhere, Geoffrey Lean ('New Poison Threat to Japan', *Observer*, 22.6.80) states: 'More than 300 have died and nearly 1,500 have been officially recognised as having the disease. A further 6,000 claim they have it.'

15. The link between Minemata disease and the mercury discharged in Chisso's industrial waste was not made until 1962 (Watanuki, *op.cit.* 1978, p.5). Although it was quickly realised that contaminated fish were responsible for the disease, mercury was not initially suspected as the pollutant. Even when it was singled out as the culprit (in 1959), investigators failed to pin the source down to Chisso. One reason, perhaps, was that Chisso failed to report that it was discharging mercury in its wastes (Tucker, *op.cit.* 1972, p.26). Another, undoubtedly, was that the mercury discharged from Chisso (when finally analysed) was in an *inorganic* form: that found in the contaminated fish and shellfish was dimethyl mercury, an *organic* and extremely toxic form of the metal. It was not until later that it was discovered that inorganic mercury was being converted to dimethyl mercury by the marine ecosystem. It has also been alleged that 'company doctors concealed important experimental data on cats which showed that

the disease originated from factory waste water' (Watanuki, *op.cit.* 1978, p.5).

16. Although the company paid token damages to Minemata victims (£100 to adults, £30 to children) it consistently denied responsibility for the disaster. Indeed, those who received compensation did so only after signing a document 'which precluded all action for further compensation even if "at some future time the Minemata disease is proven to be the result of waste from the plant" '. (Tucker, *op.cit.* 1972, pp.44-45).

17. S. Sterrett and C.A. Boss, 'Careless Kepone', *Environment*, Vol. 19, No.2, March 1977, p.34. Concentration of Kepone 'in edible tissues of most fish and estuarine fin fish and shellfish ranged from 0.1 to 1 part per million (ppm)'. The 'safe' limit set by the US Food and Drug Administration is 0.1 ppm.

18. Congressional Research Service, *Background Material Requested for Use in the Consideration of H.R. 7040, A Bill requiring Disclosure of Certain Information by Business Entities*, Library of Congress, Washington D.C., 1980, p.21: F. Sterrett and C. Boss (*op.cit.* 1977, p.31).

19. Congressional Research Service, *op.cit.* 1980, pp.21-22.

20. F. Sherrett and C. Boss, *op.cit.* 1977, p.31. Concentrations of Kepone ranged from 0.02 to 0.3 ppm.

21. E. Eckholm, *Down to Earth*, Pluto, London, 1982, p.82.

22. Clive Cookson, 'The Spoiling of America', *New Scientist*, 21.6.79, p.1016. David Dickson ('Lessons of Love Canal Prompt Clean-Up', *Ambio*, Vol. 11, No.1, 1982, p.48) gives a figure of between $28 and $55 billion for cleaning up all of America's hazardous waste sites.

23. Marjorie Sun, 'EPA Relaxes Hazardous Waste Rules', *Science*, Vol. 216, 16.4.82, pp. 275-276.

24. J. Carvel, 'Row over Toxic Plan', *Guardian*, 24.1.81 for a critique of Britain's new regulations, see: 'Joint Brief on Regulations Laid Before Parliament' SO NO. 1709/1980 under Section 17 of Control of Pollution Act 1974, Association of County Councils, London, 1981.

25. B.D. David (Executive Vice-President, Industrial Chemicals Group, Hooker Chemical Company), statement before Committee on Interstate and Foreign Commerce; Subcommittee on Oversight and Investigations, *Hearings on Hazardous Waste Disposal*, (Part I), US House of Representatives (96th Congress, 1st Session) Washington D.C., 1979, pp.502-503.

26. *Hearings on Hazardous Waste Disposal* (Part 1). Committee on Interstate and Foreign Commerce; Subcommittee on Oversight and Investigations, US House of Representatives, (96th Congress, 1st Session), Washington D.C., 1979, p.502. (Hereafter referred to as: '*Hearings on Hazardous Waste Disposal* (Part I) 1979.)

27. Ibid. pp. 651-652.

28. I. Molotsky, 'A Love Canal Warning No-one can Recall', *New York Times*, 14.4.79: Congressional Research Service, *op.cit.* 1980, p.31.

29. *Hearings on Hazardous Waste Disposal*, (Part I) *op.cit.* 1979, pp.651-

652. It should be noted, however, that there is an addendum to the memo: 'Since writing this memo F.L. Bryant has discussed this matter with Mr Salacruse, attorney for the School Board'.

30. Michael Brown, *Laying Waste: The Poisoning of America by Toxic Chemicals*, Pantheon, New York, 1980, p.25-26. Undoubtedly the residents of Love Canal owe much to the dedication of Michael Brown, the journalist who first broke the story. He singly refused to be bullied into silence.

31. R. Whalen, *Love Canal – Public Health Time Bomb*, Special Report to the Governor and Legislature, New York State Department of Health, 1978, p.4.

32. T.H. Maugh II, 'Toxic Waste Disposal a Growing Problem?' *Science*, Vol. 204, 25.5.79, p.820.

33. R. Whalen, *op.cit.* 1978, p.14.

34. T.H. Maugh II, *op.cit.* 25.5.79, p.820.

35. *Hazardous Waste Disposal* (Part I), *op.cit.* 1979, pp.63-64.

36. Ibid. p.80.

37. M. Brown, *op.cit.* p.57.

38. J. Raloff, 'Disaster on 99th Street', *New Scientist*, 19.6.80, p.229.

39. I. Molotsky, 'Damage to Chromosomes Found in Love Canal Tests', *New York Times*, 16.5.80.

40. J. Raloff, *op.cit.* 19.6.80, p.300.

41. J. Raloff, 'The Human Cost of Love Canal', *New Scientist*, 3.7.80.

42. M. Brown, *op.cit.* 1980, p.62.

43. Ibid. p.69.

44. 'Dioxin in the Great Lakes', *New Scientist*, 15.1.81. Levels of dioxin in herring gulls' eggs in Lake Ontario were as high as 64 parts per trillion. 'Levels found in eggs that had been refrigerated in 1971 and analysed (in 1980) . . . showed levels of 800 ppt.' According to *New Scientist*, Douglas Hallet of the Canadian Wildlife Service performed the survey of herring gulls' eggs and concluded in a paper to the government that waste disposal or "catastrophic accidents" during 2,4,5,-T manufacture by Hooker Chemicals at Niagara Falls, is the most likely source of Lake Ontario's dioxins.'

45. M. Brown, *op.cit.* 1981, p.74. Also: *Hazardous Waste Disposal* (Part I) *op.cit.* 1979, p.193 ff.

46. J. Raloff, *op.cit.* 19.6.80, p.300.

47. R.J. Smith, 'Love Canal Study Attracts Criticism', *Science*, Vol. 217, 20.8.82, p.714.

48. R.J. Smith, 'The Risks of Living Near Love Canal', *Science*, Vol. 217, 27.8.82, p.808.

49. N. Haneson, 'Is Love Canal Safe for People Again?' *New Scientist*, 22.7.82.

50. R.J. Smith, 'The Risks of Living Near Love Canal', *Science*, Vol. 217, 27.8.82.

51. News Release, Occidental International Oil, New York, 14.7.82.

52. T.H. Maugh II, 'Toxic Waste Disposal a Growing Problem', *Science*, Vol. 204, 25.5.79.

53. *Oversight: Resource Conservation and Recovery Act*, Committee on Interstate and Foreign Commerce, House of Representatives 95-183, Washington D.C., 1978, p.1. (Hereinafter referred to as Oversight RCRA).

54. Oversight RCRA, *op.cit.* 1978, pp.1-3.

55. Marjorie Sun, 'EPA Relaxes Hazardous Waste Rules', *Science*, Vol. 216, 16.4.82, p.275.

56. Ibid. p.275.

57. Ibid. p.275.

58. H.B. Kaufman, Testimony before Oversight RCRA, *op.cit.* 1978, p.305.

59. Ibid. pp.312-313.

60. Ibid. p.306

61. Ibid. p.317; memo dated 16.5.78.

62. Ibid. p.318; memo dated 14.4.78.

63. Ibid. pp.320-321, brief dated 2.10.78.

64. G. Miller, Statement before Subcommittee on Crime of the House Judiciary Committee, H.R. 4973, Washington D.C., 1980. All the memoranda referred to in this incident appear in his testimony.

65. Oversight RCRA, *op.cit.* 1978, pp.90-305.

66. Ibid. pp.157-163.

67. Ibid. pp.111,219.

68. Ibid. p.215.

69. Ibid. p.215.

70. Ibid. p.217.

71. Ibid. p.218.

72. Ibid. p.349.

73. Ibid. p.306.

74. Ibid. p.348.

75. Ibid. p.216.

76. Ibid. pp. 296,301.

77. Ibid. p.221.

78. D. Dickson, 'Lessons of Love Canal Prompt Clean-Up', *Ambio*, Vol. 11, No. 1, 1982, p.48.

79. Interview with Anthony Fagin, London, 1979.

80. House of Lords Select Committee on Science and Technology, *Hazardous Waste Disposal*, Vol. 1 (Report), HMSO, London, 1981. (Hereinafter referred to as House of Lords Select Committee.)

81. Ibid. p.26.

82. Ibid. pp.71-78.

83. Ibid. p.39.

84. Ibid. p.26: See also, Fred Pearce and Catherine Caufield, 'Toxic Waste: the political connections', *New Scientist,* 14.5.81, p.410.

85. House of Lords Select Committee, *op.cit.* 1981, p.5.

86. *The Disposal of Toxic Waste*, Report by the Key Committee, HMSO, London, 1970.

87. House of Lords' Select Committee, *op.cit.* 1981, p.7.

88. Brian Price, 'Buried but not dead', *Guardian*, 21.1.81.

89. The Disposal of Toxic Waste, Report by the Key Committee, HMSO, London, 1970.

90. 'Pollution costs firm over £1000', *Manchester Evening News*, 15.7.70.

91. Fred Pearce, 'Toxic Waste: The Cowboys are Back in Business', *New Scientist*, 11.3.82., p.626.

92. James Lewis, 'Spray Could be Causing Miscarriages', *Guardian*, 18.6.78: 'Forestry Commission Stops Dumping of Weed-killer Drums', *Guardian*, 26.11.79.

93. 'Fines for West Midland Waste-disposal Firms', *Municipal Engineering*, 8.11.77.

94. *Clyde River Purification Board Report*, 1978, pp.74-75.

95. *Birmingham Post*, 8.1.80: *Evening Mail*, 10.1.80: *Express and Star*, 8.1.80, 9.1.80.

96. Ewan Clarkson, 'The Bottomless Pit', *Guardian*, 28.11.79.

97. M.R. Hawkins, *Report by the Devon County Engineer on Higher Kiln Quarry, Bampton*, 22.7.77, p.3. The company wanted to dump up to 7 million gallons more liquid waste and another 10,000 tons of solids a year. The list of chemicals submitted for dumping approval ranged from pharmaceuticals to 'unidentified chemicals' and 'other industrial waste'.

98. 'DOE refuses help with Bubbling Cauldron', *Municipal Engineering*, 5.7.77: A.Q. Khan, *Investigation and Treatment at Ravensfield Tip*, 1979, pp.3 and 5. It has since cost Yorkshire County Council over £250,000 to excavate the tip and neutralise the acid tars. (See also: Pearce and Caufield, *op.cit.* 14.5.81, p.410.)

99. Catherine Caufield and Fred Pearce, 'An Overburden of Toxic Waste', *New Scientist*, 7.5.81, p.344.

100. Ibid. pp.344-346.

101. 'Tip Hazard', *New Scientist*, 7.1.82, p.8.

102. Caufield and Pearce, *op.cit.* 7.5.81, p.346.

103. Ibid. p.346.

104. 'Toxic Tip Closed', *New Scientist*, 4.2.82, p.296.

105. *The Disposal of Toxic Waste*, Report by the Key Committee, HMSO, London, 1970.

106. *The Behaviour of Hazardous Waste in Landfill*, Institute of Geological Sciences, HMSO, 1978 (Summary and Conclusions).

107. 'Howell Names 53 Danger Waste Tips', *Guardian*, 30.4.75.

108. Interview with Brian Cope, Birmingham, 1980. See also: Brian Cope, *The Saturated Sponge*, A Teach-in Presentation to Basildon District Council, 25.3.80. Cope argues that the very nature of landfill makes pollution unavoidable. He points out that landfill operates on the same

principle as a sponge: toxic wastes are poured on domestic refuse, which soaks them up and then breaks them down as it degrades. The success of the operation depends on how rapidly the 'sponge' becomes saturated because, once saturated, the 'sponge' can no longer soak up new wastes and they migrate rapidly to other areas outside the tip.

109. Bob Keen, 'Toxic Substances: Wasted Opportunities', *New Scientist*, 15.12.77, p.689.

110. 'Waste Authorities Face "Dilute and Disperse" Pressure', *New Civil Engineer*, 27.1.77, p.35.

111. Ibid. p.35.

112. R. Aspinwall, Government Inspectors Report on Pitsea Planning Application, November 1978, p.45: A.W. Davies (Anglian Water Authority), Government Inspectors Report on Pitsea Planning Application, November 1978, p.54.

113. Letter from J.C. Rosser, Basildon Town Council, to Ellison and Co., Solicitors to Redland-Purle, 10.11.78.

114. House of Lords Select Committee, *op.cit.* 1981, p.14.

115. Ibid. p.14.

116. Ibid. p.14.

117. Ibid. p.40.

118. Ibid. p.12.

119. Ibid. p.40.

120. Pearce and Caufield, *op.cit.* 14.5.81, pp.409-410.

121. Ibid. p.409.

122. House of Lords Select Committee, *op.cit.* 1981, p.31.

123. Ibid. p.31. The rigid definition of toxicity makes avoidance by mixing wastes possible.

124. Fred Pearce, *op.cit.* 11.3.82, p.628.

125. 'Econotes', *Audubon*, Spring 1978.

126. Press Release, Office of New Jersey's Attorney-General, 13.2.77, pp.2-3.

127. Press Release, Office of New Jersey's Attorney-General, 22.9.77, p.1.

128. A. Schneider, 'Gypsy Trucks Carry Poisonous Chemicals into Forests and Fields', *Washington Post,* 11.4.80.

Chapter 3: Radiation: How Low Can You Get?

1. C. Lushbaugh, Statement before Subcommittee on Health and the Environment of the Committee on Interstate and Foreign Commerce; *Effect of Radiation on Human Health*, US House of Representatives, Washington D.C., 1978, p.790 (hereafter: *Effect of Radiation on Human Health*).

2. P. Bunyard, 'Radiation Risks, how low can one get?' *New Ecologist*, September 1978. See also, P. Bunyard, *Nuclear Britain*, New English Libary, London, 1981.

3. *Effects of Radiation on Human Health*, *op.cit.* 1978, p.5. (Testimony of Karl Z. Morgan.)

4. J. Garrison and C. Ryle, *Low-Dose Radiation and ICRP 26,* Information Service on Radiation and Health, Cambridge 1979.

5. *Health Effects of Ionizing Radiation,* Vols. 1 and 2. Joint Hearings of the Committee on Interstate and Foreign Commerce of the US House of Representatives and the Labour and Human Resources Committee of the US Senate, Washington D.C., 1979. Serial No. 96-41.

6. *US News and World Report*, 'Atomic Test Toll, A Generation Later', 30.4.79.

7. Joyce Eggington, 'Deadly Dust that Kills by Stealth', *Observer,* 10.8.80.

8. Interview with veteran attending Citizens' Hearings on Radiation Victims, Washington D.C., 1980.

9. *Effects of Radiation on Human Health, op.cit.* 1979, p.53.

10. D. Dickson, 'A-Bomb Tests Linked to Rise in Childhood Leukaemia', *Nature*, 8.2.79.

11. Giff Johnson, 'Nuclear Legacy', *Oceans*, January 1980.

12. Ibid.

13. Press Release, Nevada Test Organisation, Office of Information 24.8.57. Reproduced in *Effects of Radiation on Human Health, op.cit.* 1978, p.62.

14. *Effects of Radiation on Human Health, op.cit.* 1978, p.197 ff.

15. Ibid. pp.214-215.

16. *Health Effects of Ionizing Radiation,* Vols. 1 and 2., *op.cit.* 1979.

17. D. Dickson, *op.cit.* 1979.

18. *Health Effects of Ionizing Radiation, op.cit.* 1979, pp.31-33.

19. Ibid. pp.18, 28-29, 98-99.

20. In August 1982, Judge A. Sherman Christenson overthrew his own verdict in a 1956 trial which had found against some Utah sheep farmer who had alleged that their sheep had been damaged by radiation from the early Nevada Tests. Judge Sherman's decision was taken because he felt the US government had 'perpetrated a fraud on the court' by suppressing evidence and pressurising witnesses. (See: Joyce Eggington, 'Billions Sought to Compensate A-test victims', *Observer,* 19.8.82.)

21. *Interagency Task Force on Low Dose Radiation*, Washington D.C., 1979.

22. Testimony presented before Citizens Hearings on Radiation Victims, Washington D.C., 1980.

23. I. Bross, Testimony on Reauthorisation for Chairman Henry Waxman's Subcommittee, Washington D.C., 1980.

24. In this respect it is interesting to note the contents of a memo in 1977 to the US Deputy Assistant Secretary of Defense on the subject of nuclear testing: 'there has been considerable media exposure on this matter to date . . . . If we do not respond appropriately, we can expect to have the same

kind of adverse publicity as that experienced in regard to the asbestos problem.' (*Effects of Radiation on Human Health, op.cit.* 1978, p.217).

25. Testimony of Mrs Harding before Citizens Hearing on Radiation Victims, Washington D.C., 1980.

26. Pierre Fruhling, 'Uranium Killed Joe Harding', Citizens Hearing on Radiation Victims, Washington D.C., 1980. All quotes from Joe Harding come from this article.

27. J. Garrison and C. Ryle, *op.cit.* 1979.

28. *Effects of Radiation on Health, op.cit.* 1978, p.71 ff. (Testimony of Dr Tamplin.)

29. *Effects of Radiation on Health, op.cit.* 1978, p.73.

30. Interview with I. Bross, Buffalo, 1980.

31. J. Garrison and C. Ryle, *op.cit.* 1979.

32. Lee Torrey, 'Radiation Haunts Shipyard Workers', *New Scientist,* 16.3.78.

33. 'Scientist Changes Cover-Up', *Not Man Apart*, March, 1979.

34. The documents are reproduced in *Effects of Radiation on Health, op.cit.* 1978. See in particular, p.523 ff. (Testimony and Statement of Thomas F. Mancuso.)

35. Letter from Professor William Schull to Leonard Sagan, AEC Contract Officer for the Health and Mortality Study, 8.11.67.

36. Letter from Professor Brian MacMahon to Leonard Sagan, 13.11.67.

37. Memorandum from John Totter to S.G. English, 28.2.72.

38. See *Effects of Radiation on Human Health, op.cit.* 1978, pp.497-501 for details of Milham's study.

39. Draft note to Files on Milham/Mancuso Occupational Radiation Exposure Studies, R.P. Fasulo, 1.7.75.

40. Draft Press Release, AEC, 1974.

41. Interview with Mancuso, Pittsburg, 1980. See Also Mancuso's testimony, *Effects of Radiation on Human Health, op.cit.* 1978.

42. R. Pollock, 'Uncovering Nuclear Cancer', *In These Times*, March 22-28, 1978.

43. *Effects of Radiation on Human Health, op.cit.* 1978, p.536.

44. Marks himself acknowledges in a memorandum that: 'Dr Mancuso's inclination is to achieve something approaching perfection in the quality of the data before starting analysis.' (*Effects of Radiation on Human Health, op.cit.* 1978, p.563.)

45. Draft Memorandum of Sidney Marks, 20.2.73.

46. *Effects of Radiation on Human Health, op.cit.* 1978.

47. Interview with Mancuso, Pittsburg, 1980. See also, *Effects of Radiation on Human Health*, p.570. In a letter to Dr Sanders, George Kneale points out that, on the basis of Sanders's analysis, 'The risk of dying was reduced by 42 per cent. This is so large as to defy belief even in the most confirmed believer in the beneficial effects of low level radiation.'

48. See P. Bunyard, *op.cit.* 1978 for further discussion of Stewart's previous research.

49. Mancuso, Stewart, Kneale, 'Radiation Exposures of Hanford Workers Dying of Cancer and Other Causes', *Health Physics* 33(S), 1977. Also: Mancuso, Stewart and Kneale, *Reanalysis of the Data Relating to the Hanford Study*, paper presented at International Symposium on Late Biological Effects of Ionizing Radiation, Vienna, 1978.

50. Ibid. See also, Harvey Wasserman and Norman Solomon, *Killing our Own,* Delta, USA, 1982, p.143: 'There were indications of a 5 to 7 per cent excess in radiation cancer deaths among Hanford workers at exposure levels as much as thirty times *below* what had been considered safe.'

51. P. Bunyard, *op.cit.* 1978.

52. Interview with Stewart, Birmingham, 1978 and 1980.

53. P. Bunyard, E. Goldsmith and N. Hildyard, *Reprocessing the Truth,* Supplement to *New Ecologist*, April 1978.

Chapter 4: The Truth About Microwaves

1. For a full discussion of the manner in which the 10 milliwatt standard was set, see Paul Brodeur, *The Zapping of America: Microwaves, their deadly risk and the cover-up*, Norton, New York, 1978, chapters 1-2.

2. *Report of the Electromagnetic Radiation Advisory Council of the White House Office of Telecommunication Policy*, OTP-ERMAC, Washington D.C., 1971. 'Radiation emanating from radar, television, communications systems and microwave ovens . . . permeates the modern environment. In the decades ahead, man may enter an era of energy pollution of the environment comparable to the chemical pollution of today.' Quoted in 'Electromagnetic smog', *Common Weal Research Publications*, Vol. 1 No. 9, Bolinas, California, March 1978, p.1.

3. Lowell Ponte, 'The Menace of Electrical Smog' *Reader's Digest,* January 1980, p.66.

4. P. Brodeur, *op.cit.* 1978, p.60.

5. Ibid. p.60.

6. Ibid. p.61.

7. Ibid. p.61.

8. Ibid. p.61.

9. Ibid. p.61.

10. Ibid, see in particular chapter 7, p.95 ff. Lowell Ponte (*op.cit.* 1980, p.67) notes: 'Embassy personnel were not informed of the irradiation. Instead they were asked to give blood samples to "test for a disease in Moscow's water". The tests revealed that a third had white blood-cell counts almost 50 per cent higher than normal – often a symptom of severe infection and also a characteristic of leukaemia.'

11. Brodeur, *op.cit.* 1978, p.56.

12. Ibid. pp.57-59.

13. Ibid. p.59.
14. Ibid. p.63.
15. Ibid. p.63.
16. Ibid. p.63.
17. Ibid. pp.63-64.
18. *Common Weal Research Publications, op.cit.* p.4.
19. Ibid. p.6.
20. Susan Schiefelbein, 'The Invisible Threat; the Stifled Story of Electric Waves', *Saturday Review*, 15.9.79, p.17.
21. Brodeur (*op.cit.* 1978), p.44) comments: 'Professor Schwan (also pointed out) that investigators who tried to acquire information about microwave injuries were encountering difficulties from employers, and he deplored a tendency on the part of the military and industry "to dismiss the possibilities of microwave-induced damage in order to avoid legal and compensation problems". After defending the 10-milliwatt standard as "the best we can formulate on the basis of presently available knowledge", he admitted that it had been "crudely set" and "badly needs refinement".'
22. Discussing the Russian Studies, Suskind observed: 'We cannot very well dismiss a whole body of scientific literature just because it is Russian', (Brodeur, *op.cit.* 1978, p.43).
23. Brodeur, *op.cit.* 1978, pp.35-38. Another reason for the Russian evidence being dismissed, says Brodeur, was that: 'Translations of the Russian experiments were often grossly inaccurate.' (p.39).
24. Ibid. 1978.
25. Ibid. 1978.
26. Milton Zaret, Testimony before Senate Committee on Commerce, Science and Transport, *Hearings on Radiation Control for Safety and Health,* US Senate, Washington D.C., 1973 (93-24) pp.101-102.
27. Ibid. p.102.
28. Susan Schiefelbein, *op.cit.* 1979, p.18.
29. Peter Gwynne, 'The Zap Flap', *Newsweek*, 17.7.78, p.43.
30. Keith Hindley, 'Death by Microwave', *Sunday Times*, 9.8.81.
31. Pearce Wright, 'Microwave Accusation Touches Raw Nerve', *The Times*, 9.9.81.
32. For an excellent discussion of the Moscow incident, see P. Brodeur, *op.cit.* 1978, p.94 ff; see also *Common Weal Research Publications, op.cit.* 1978, p.6; and *Microwave Irradiation of the US Embassy in Moscow*, Committee on Commerce, Science, and Transportation, US Senate, Washington D.C., 1979, p.12.
33. Susan Schiefelbein, *op.cit.* 1979, p.18
34. Susan Schiefelbein, *op.cit.* 1979, p.18; *Common Weal Research Publications, op.cit.* 1978, p.6.
35. Ibid. 1978.
37. *Microwave Irradiation of the US Embassy in Moscow*, Committee on Commerce, Science and Transportation, US Senate, Washington D.C.,

1979, p.4. The Study also noted, however, 'that 38 per cent of the control subjects (based on corresponding analysis of blood samples taken before assignment of those subjects to the Moscow Embassy) fell into that risk classification.' (p.5).

37. P. Brodeur, *op.cit.* 1978, p.94 ff; *Common Weal Research Publications*, *op.cit.* 1978, p.6.

38. S. Schiefelbein, *op.cit.* 1979, p.17.

39. Ibid. p.17. In addition to citing Project Pandora, the State Department also commissioned an epidemiological study of some 4,000 former employees of the Moscow Embassy. The study, conducted by Dr Abraham Lilienfeld of Johns Hopkins University, came to the conclusion that embassy employees had not 'encountered health hazards traceable to their exposure.' The study had been designed by the State Department, which also supplied all the information. 'While government officials tout this study as cause for great relief – a vindication of microwaves – Lilienfeld himself calls for caution in the interpretation of his results,' reports Schiefelbein. 'He says he "would not use the word *reassuring* to describe the report. Since the latency period of cancer can be as long as 20 years, and since the people who had the highest doses were exposed as late as 1977, there has been little follow up".' (pp.17-18).

40. P. Brodeur, *op.cit.* 1978.

41. P. Brodeur, *op.cit.* 1978, p.90.

42. Ibid. p.91. Comments Brodeur: 'Almost 10 per cent of the fathers of children with Down's syndrome reported "intimate contact with radar both in and outside of the armed forces" compared to slightly more than 3 per cent of the fathers in the control group.' It should be noted, however, that a second Johns Hopkins Study, carried out a decade later, did not find any statistically significant relationship between Down's syndrome and the exposure of parents to radar. But, as Brodeur points out: '(The Study) does . . . suggest that men exposed to the emanation of radar have a significant increase in the number of chromosomal abnormalities in their blood – a finding that, since chromosomal abnormalities can cause birth defects, leaves the whole question of the genetic effects of microwave radiation in human beings open to further investigation.' (p.92).

43. Ibid. 1978.

44. Ibid. 1978.

45. Ibid. 1978.

46. Interview with Andrew Marino, Syracuse, New York 1980. Also: Andrew A. Marino and Robert O. Becker, 'High Voltage Lines, Hazard at a Distance', *Environment*, November 1978, p.7.

47. Dr Robert O. Becker, Testimony before State of New York Public Service Commission, (Cases 26529 and 26559 – *Common Record Hearings on Health and Safety of 765 kv. Transmission Lines*) Albany, New York, 1977.

48. Becker and Marino, 'Electromagnetic Pollution', *The Sciences,*

January 1978, p.15: See also, Louise B. Young, 'Danger: High Voltage', *Environment*, May 1978, p.37.

49. Becker and Marino, *op.cit.* January 1978, p.15.

50. A.A. Marino, Testimony, 1977. At the New York hearings, Marino's work on both rats and mice came in for much criticism. The State of New York Public Service Commission in its summing up argued that the rat experiments 'indicate that electric fields may cause stress but (are) not conclusive'; the mice studies were described as 'excellent' and it was accepted that they showed that 'ELF fields can cause adverse biological effects.' Initial Brief, *Cases 26529 and 26559 – Common Record Hearings on Health and Safety of 765 kv. Transmission Lines,* Albany, New York 1977, pp.11 ff and 27 ff.

51. A. Marino, Testimony, *op.cit.* 1977.

52. Ibid.

53. R.O. Becker, Testimony, *op.cit.* 1977. In his testimony Marino went further; 'It is . . . evident that to permit chronic human exposure at or near electric field strengths which have produced biological effects in test animals would be cruel, barbaric and inhumane.' (*Amicus Curiae Brief,* p.28).

54. Louise B. Young, *op.cit.* 1978, p.19: V.P. Korobkova, Yu.A. Morozov, MD, Stolarov and Yu.A. Yakup, *Influence of the Electric Field in 500 and 750 kv. Switchyards on Maintenance Staff and Means for its Protection,* International Conference on Large High Tension Electric Systems (CIGRE), Paris, Aug-Sep 1972.

55. Louise B. Young, *Power over People*, Oxford, 1977.

56. L.B. Young, *op.cit.* 1978, p.19.

57. For details of these and other experiments, see A. Marino, *Testimony*, *op.cit.* 1977, (in particular Exhibit C-5); Louise B. Young, *op.cit.* 1978; Becker and Marino, *op.cit.* November 1978, pp.11-12. At the New York public hearings on the safety of 765 kv. transmission lines, Marino accused the utility company which had applied to build the transmission line of having 'dirty hands with regard to the Soviet scientific literature'. He noted, 'As far back as 1970, the open scientific literature of the Soviet Union contained more than 100 reports of the biological effects of ELF fields and since that time the scope of the Soviet research effort has increased.' Yet, Marino continued, 'almost no acceptable Soviet scientific information on the biological effects of ELF fields is openly available in the United States'. Since the Russians have always been willing to share their data, Mario concluded that there were only two explanations for the unavailability of Russian studies in the US; either 'the Soviets have never been requested to tender information'; or 'the Soviets have tendered the information but the utility companies . . . have not made it generally available'. Finally, he commented: 'Withholding information or failing to obtain it where there was a clear duty to do so is wrongdoing.' (See A. Marino, *Amicus Curiae Brief,* pp.30-31.)

59. Louise B. Young, *op.cit.* 1978, p.19.

60. Interview with Marino, Syracuse, New York, 1980; Susan Schiefelbein, *op.cit.* 1979, p.18.

61. S. Schiefelbein, *op.cit.* 1979, p.18.

62. *Proceedings of the Ad Hoc Committee for the Review of Biomedical and Ecological Effects of ELF radiation*, US Department of the Navy, Bureau of Medicine and Surgery, 1973, p.21.

63. R.O. Becker, Letter to Commissioner Henry Diamond, 10.12.73.

64. Interview with A. Marino, Syracuse, New York, 1980.

65. A. Marino, *Amicus Curiae Brief on Exceptions, State of New York Public Service Commission, (Cases 26529 and 26559) – Common Record Hearings on Health and Safety of 765 kv. Transmission Lines)* Albany, New York, 1978, pp.4-5.

66. S. Schiefelbein, *op.cit.* 1979, p.19.

67. A. Marino, *Amicus Curiae Brief on Exceptions, op.cit.* 1978, pp.6-8.

68. According to Schiefelbein (*op.cit.* 1979, p.19) the Navy's decision to reproduce the Sanguine study resulted largely because Senator Gaylor Nelson of Wisconsin (where the project was to be built) obtained a copy of the Tyler report. As Schiefelbein reports: 'Nelson issued a press release stating that the Navy had apparently "kept the wraps on the existence of this report because it contains the very first scientific evidence that Sanguine would have an adverse environmental impact".' (p.19.).

69. S. Schiefelbein, *op.cit.* 1979, p.19: Interview with Marino, Syracuse, New York, 1980.

70. S. Schiefelbein, *op.cit.* 1979, p.19.

71. T.R. Mathias and H.L. Colbeth, *Recommended Decision of the Administrative Law Judges on the Health and Safety Effects of 765 kv. Transmission Lines,* State of New York Public Service Commission, Albany, New York, 1978, p.136.

72. *Opinion and Order Determining Health and Safety Issues, Imposing Operating Conditions and Authorizing, in Case 26529, Operation Pursuant to Conditions*, State of New York Public Service Commission, p.12 and p.71 ff.

73. Ibid. p.39.

74. S. Schiefelbein, *op.cit.* 1979, p.20.

75. Interview with Hilary Bacon, 1980.

76. Ibid. See also Simon Best: 'Pylon Power', *Doctor*, 19.3.81, p.42. Best notes: 'In 1978, five people experienced black-outs beneath the Fishpond lines. (But) it was not until later at a public inquiry that the Fishpond residents learnt for the first time that voltage on one arm of the Fishpond line had been increased from 132 to 345 kilovolts at the time the first black-out was reported.' Bacon, in her testimony at Haddington, 1982, reports the increase to have been from 275 to 345 kilovolts. (H. Bacon, 'Proof of evidence for Haddington Public Inquiry into the Siting of Overhead High-voltage Transmission lines from Torness Nuclear Power Station'.

Haddington, April 1982, p.14).

77. Interview with Bacon, Fishpond 1980. See also, H. Bacon, 'Proof of Evidence', *op.cit.* 1982, p.9 and enclosures 19 and 20.

78. See, for instance, J. Bonnell, 'Proof of Evidence before Innsworth Public Inquiry', Gloucester, 1978, pp. 2,5.

79. P. Brodeur, *op.cit.* 1978.

80. J. Bonnell, *op.cit.* 1978, p.2.

81. Becker and Marino, *op.cit.* November 1978, p.8.

82. The studies cited by Bonnell were: T.P. Asanova *et al.* 'Health Condition of Workers Exposed to an Electrical Field of 400-500 kilovolts Open Distribution Installations', Labour, Hygiene and Occupational Diseases, No.5, 1966, pp.72-76: T.E. Sazanova: 'The Physiological Effects of Work in the Vicinity of 400 kilovolt and 500 kilovolt Outdoor Installations', *Naucnye Raboty Institutov Ohrany Truda*, VCSPS No.46, 1967, pp.34-39. Korobkova *et al*: 'Influence of the Electric Field in 500 and 750 kilovolt Switchyards on Maintenance Staff and Means for its Protection', CIGRE paper 23-06, 1972. Krivova *et al,* 'The Influence of an Electric Field of Commercial Frequency and Discharges on the Human Organism'. Both the latter papers are cited by Bonnell as 'referred to in "Biological Effects of High Voltage Electric Fields", ERPI 38-1, Final Report, November 1975'. Bonnell gives no other source for the Krivova paper.

83. J. Bonnell, *op.cit.* 1978, p.2.

84. Ibid. p.5.

85. Ibid. p.5.

86. Ibid. pp. 2-3.

87. Ibid. p.2. The references Bonnell cited were: *Revue Generale de L'Electricité,* Numero Special, July 1976. W.B. Kouwenhoven *et al.* Medical Evaluation of Men Working in A/C Electric Fields', Transactions 1 EEE PAS, Vol. 86, No.4, April 1967, p.507. Singlewald and Kouwenhoven 'Medical Follow-up Study of High Voltage Linemen Working in A/C Electric Fields', Transactions 1, EEE PAS Vol. 92, No. 4, July 1973, p.1307.

88. J. Bonnell, *op.cit.* 1978, p.3.

89. Ibid. p.3. para.8.

90. Ibid. p.3. para.10.

91. Ibid. p.3. para.10.

92. Martin Weitz, 'Power over People: Mrs Bacon vs CEGB', *New Statesman,* 17.11.78.

93. Ibid.

94. H. Bacon, *op.cit.* 1982, p.10 and passim.

95. Martin Weitz, *op.cit.* 1978: Testimony of Dr David Smith at Innsworth inquiry, Gloucester, 1978.

96. Ibid.

97. H. Bacon, *op.cit.* 1982, p.12.

98. Martin Weitz, *op.cit.* 1978.

99. Interview with H. Bacon, Fishpond, 1980.

100. Correspondence between Hawkins and Bacon, 1978-79.

101. H. Bacon, *op.cit.* 1982, p.14.

102. J. Bonnell, *op.cit.* 1978, p.5.

103. Staff's Initial Brief, Cases 26529 and 26559 – Common Record Hearing on Health and Safety of 765 kilovolt Transmission Lines, State of New York Public Service Commission, Albany, 1977.

104. State of New York Public Service Commission, *Opinion and Order Determining Health and Safety Issues, imposing operating conditions and authorizing in Case 26529, operation pursuant to those conditions,* Albany, 1978, p.12.

105. Martin Weitz, *op.cit.* 1978.

106. J. Bonnell, *op.cit.* 1978, p.4. para.17.

107. See record of Innsworth Inquiry, Gloucester, 1978.

108. Interview with H. Bacon, Fishpond, 1980. H. Bacon, *op.cit.* 1982, pp.12-13.

119. H. Bacon, *op.cit.* 1982, p.15.

110. H. Bacon, *op.cit.* 1982, p.13. See also record of Innsworth Inquiry, Gloucester, 1978.

111. *Guardian*, 23.6.1981.

112. Interview with H. Bacon, Fishpond, 1982.

113. See record of Haddington Inquiry, Haddington, East Lothian, 1982.

114. *British Medical Journal*, Vol. 281, p.117.

115. J. Bonnell *et al. Les Champs Electriques et Magnetiques et L'Homme,* General World Health Organisation, 1979. (CM-22.12.1979-101.47).

116. Letter quoted by H. Bacon at Haddington inquiry, 1982.

117. Ibid.

118. Interview with H. Bacon, Fishpond, 1982.

119. Details of these blackouts are given in a letter Bacon wrote to Jim Spicer, MP, on 11 June, 1982.

120. Andrew Veitch, 'Shocking Tale of Addiction in a Grid', *Guardian*, 21.4.82.

121. Ibid.

122. Interview with H. Bacon, 1982.

123. The revised version of this chapter was completed in December 1982.

124. Report of Inspectors, Public Inquiry into Walham-Springs 400 kilovolt Line, 1980.

125. Ibid. See also: David Mellor, letter to Jim Spencer, 12.11.82.

126. In the first edition of *Cover-Up* I stated: 'For its part, the CEGB had carried out no research into the health hazards of low-frequency electrical fields.' When this statement was repeated in a review, Brian S. Murray, a CEGB Regional Public Relations Officer, wrote to a local newspaper drawing attention 'to some inaccuracies' in *Cover-Up*. 'The CEGB,' he

wrote, 'is well aware of its responsibilities of ensuring that any adverse effects its operations may have on its staff, the general public and the environment are controlled. To this end, the Board is carrying out its own research programme and assisting other British authorities who are undertaking similar investigations.' Such investigations are now being carried out. However, as mentioned in the text, the public has yet to see the results.

127. Andrew Veitch, *op.cit.* 21.4.82.
128. Ibid.
129. David Mellor, *op.cit.* 12.11.82.
130. See for example, Marie Rachmanis *et al*, 'Relationships Between Suicide and the Electromagnetic Field of Overhead Power Lines' *Physiological Chemistry and Physics*, Vol.II, no.5, 1979, p.395. S. Milham, 'Mortality from Leukaemia in Workers Exposed to Electrical and Magnetic Fields', *New England Journal of Medicine*, Vol. 307, No.4. J. Delgado et al, 'Embryological Changes Induced by Weak, Extremely Low Frequency Electromagnetic Fields' *Journal of Anatomy*, 1982, Vol. 3, No. 134, pp.533-551.
131. BBC Radio 4 'Today' Programme, 15.11.82.
132. BBC Radio 4 'Checkpoint', 21.9.78.
133. P. Brodeur, *op.cit.* 1978.
134. Martin Weitz, *op.cit.* 1978.
135. Marie Reichmanis et al, *op.cit.*
136. 'Microwave Safety Found Lax', *Not Man Apart*, 1978.
137. Ibid.
138. Ibid.
139. Ibid.
140. P. Brodeur, *op.cit.* 1978.
142. Ibid. p.66.
142. Ibid. p.67.
143. Ibid. p.67.
144. *Common Weal Research Publications*, op.cit. 1978, p.5.
145. Ibid. p.68.
146. Ibid. p.69.
147. Ibid. p.73.
148. M. Zaret, Testimony before Senate Committee on Commerce, Science and Transport, Hearings on Radiation Control for Safety and Health, US Senate, Washington D.C., 1973 (93-24) p.104.
149. Jonathan David, 'The Microwave Boom is Stopped Cold', *Sunday Telegraph*, 28.1.79.
150. Ibid.

Chapter 5: The Pesticide Conspiracy

1. S. Epstein, *The Politics of Cancer*, Doubleday, New York, 1979, p.248.

The figure of $4 billion is a 1979 figure. Epstein points out: 'From 1950 to 1975, overall pesticide production increased from an estimated 200,000 pounds to 1.4 billion pounds.' In Britain, 'the British Agro-Chemicals Association appears to have no data at all on sales before 1974 and has only conducted two surveys of the quantities of active ingredients sold, one for 1966 and one for 1975-76. These figures suggest that sales have increased dramatically (in Britain), from about £10 million worth in 1940 to £143 million worth in 1975.' (Edward Goldsmith, 'Under Control?' *The Ecologist*, March 1980, Special Issue on Pesticides, p.102).

2. E. Goldsmith, 'Under Control?', *The Ecologist*, March 1980, Special Issue on Pesticides, p.102.

3. The Royal Commission on Environmental Pollution (7th Report, 1979) notes: 'The evidence suggests that the decline in the level of organo-chlorine compounds in the environment has not been as rapid as envisaged'. It goes on to document how eggs of sparrow-hawks (a good indicator of pollution) 'have not demonstrated a marked declined in organo-chlorine residues and in some cases there has been some evidence of increase'.

4. E. Goldsmith, *op.cit.* 1980, p.102.

5. Julian McCaul, 'Questions for an Old Friend', *Environment,* July/August 1971, p.3. McCaul stresses that the problem 'is compounded in Asian and African countries . . . since children are nursed for two or three years and DDT exposure levels may be very high'. Elsewhere (p.5) he reports on a 1971 research programme which found that the levels of DDE (a close chemical cousin of DDT) were three times higher in premature babies than in those born after the proper period of gestation. It appears that both DDT and DDE can be transported across the placental barrier to contaminate the unborn child.

6. S. Epstein (*op.cit.* 1979, p.253) points out: 'EPA monitoring programmes from 1972 to 1974 found dieldrin residues in virtually all human body fat samples analysed, with average levels of about 0.3 ppm and sometimes ranging as high as 15 ppm. Levels in blacks were about twice those in whites. These residues are relatively stable and persistent: an average of 50 per cent of initial residue levels are still present at about nine months. Further these residues are of the same order of magnitude, and in some cases greater, than levels in rodents which developed cancers after feeding with aldrin and dieldrin.'

7. The Environmental Defense Fund and Robert Boyle, *Malignant Neglect*, Vintage/Random House, New York, 1980, p.11. (Hereafter: EDF and Boyle).

8. Ibid, p.118. Epstein (*op.cit.* 1979, p.248) gives a figure of 40,000 different pesticide products. 800 formulations are now used in Britain (E. Goldsmith, *op.cit.* 1980, p.102).

9. Goldsmith, *op.cit.* 1980, p.102; Ian Nisbet, *Technology Review*, August/September 1978; EDF and Boyle, *op.cit.* pp.118-120, 134. It has been estimated that some 25 per cent of the pesticides sold in the US are

suspect carcinogens.

10. For a discussion of the political power enjoyed by the pesticide industry, see: Nisbet, *op.cit.* 1978; S. Epstein, *op.cit.* 1979, p.248 ff. (in particular p.249 note).

11. J. Warnock and J. Lewis, *The Other Face of 2,4-D,* South Okanagan Environmental Coalition, Pentacton, British Columbia, 1978, pp.1-3.

12. T. Whiteside, *The Withering Rain*, E.P. Dutton and Co., New York, 1971, p.26.

13. Ibid. p.25. Vast as this area is, it is worth noting that until 1979 (when 2,4,5-T was banned for most uses) an area of equivalent size was sprayed with 2,4,5,-T in the US *every* year (see: T. Whiteside, *The Pendulum and the Toxic Cloud*, Yale University Press, New Haven and London, 1979, p.3).

14. T. Whiteside, *op.cit.* 1971, p.26.

15. Ibid. p.36.

16. Ibid. p.37.

17. US Department of Health, Education and Welfare, *Pesticides and their Relationship to Environmental Health,* Washington D.C., 1969. (Hereafter: Mrak Commission).

18. T. Whiteside, *op.cit.* 1971, p.57. 'When the data were obtained,' reports Whiteside, 'and the White House was obliged to act, the President's science advisor publicly presented the facts in a less than candid manner, while the Department of Defense, for all practical purposes, ignored the whole business and announced its intention of going on doing what it had been doing all along.'

19. Ibid. p.40.

20. Ibid. p.39.

21. Ibid. p.40.

22. Ibid. pp.40-41.

23. S. Epstein, 'A Family Likeness', *Environment* Vol. 12, no.6, July/August 1979, p.19.

24. *Bionetics Report,* quoted in T. Whiteside, *op.cit.* 1971, p.43. At lower dose levels, 'fetal mortality was somewhat less but still quite high even when dosage was reduced to 4.6 mg/kg. The incidence of abnormal fetuses was threefold of that in controls even with the smallest dosage and shortest period used. It seems inescapable that 2,4,5,-T is teratogenic in this strain of rats (Sprague-Dawley) when given orally at the dosage schedules used here.' Later, after re-examining the Bionetics data, the Advisory Panel on Teratogenicity of Pesticides of the Department of Health, Education and Welfare, came to a similar conclusion: 'When given orally at dosages of 4.6, 10.0 and 46.6 mg/kg on days 10 through 15 of gestation, an excessive fetal mortality, up to 60 per cent at the highest dose, and a high incidence of abnormalities in the survivors was obtained. The incidence of fetuses with kidney anomalies was threefold that of controls even with the smallest dosage tested.' (Quoted in T. Whiteside, *op.cit.* 1971, p.177).

25. For further details of birth defects see J. Warnock and J. Lewis, *op.cit.* 1978.

26. Ibid. p.11-4.

27. S. Epstein, *op.cit.* 1970, p.17.

28. J. Warnock and J. Lewis, *op.cit.* 1978, p.11-4.

29. T. Whiteside, *op.cit.* 1971, p.48.

30. Ibid. p.48.

31. J. Warnock and J. Lewis, *op.cit.* 1978, p.iv-6. See also: J. Laporte, 'Effects of Dioxin Exposure', *The Lancet,* 14.5.77, p.1049. Warnock and Lewis point out that: 'Laporte notes that these figures may be understated since the Vietnamese word used to substitute for "malformation" is actually "monstrosity" and therefore tends to exclude lesser malformations.'

32. J. Warnock and J. Lewis, *op.cit.* 1978, p.iv-7. In Hanoi the incidence of Downs' Syndrome was found to be six times higher than that observed in the survivors of Hiroshima.

33. Ibid, p.11-16.

34. Mrak Commission, *op.cit.* 1979, p.18.

35. In November 1980, the *Sunday Times* reported: 'The Italian authorities are suppressing evidence on pollution by dioxin (in Seveso) . . . Pollution levels . . . are up to ten times greater than the highest values now officially registered. But the Italians are reopening roads and agricultural land in the contaminated area. The suppressed evidence means that 10,000 people could be living under a much greater risk than they have been led to believe'. (Dalbert Hallenstein, 'Seveso Danger Hushed Up', *Sunday Times,* 2.11.80.).

36. S. Epstein, *op.cit.* 1979, p.18.

37. J. Warnock and J. Lewis, *op.cit.* 1978, pp.11-8/11-9.

38. For a discussion of the levels set in the US and Britain, see: Advisory Committee on Pesticides, *Review of the Safety for Use in the UK of the Herbicide 2,4,5-T,* HMSO, London 1979-1980.

39. Ibid. p.7.

40. J. Warnock and J. Lewis, *op.cit.* 1978, pp.11-5/11-6: Doses of purified 2,4,5,-T at 100 mg/kg produced cleft palate and kidney malformations in mice. See also: S. Epstein, *op.cit.* 1970, p.18: and K.D. Courtney *et al.* 'Teratology Studies with 2,4,5,-Trichlorophenoxy-acetic acid and 2,3,7,8-Tetrachlorodibenzo-p-dioxin', *Toxicology of Applied Pharmacy* XX, 1971, p.396.

41. J. Warnock and J. Lewis, *op.cit.* 1978, p.V-9.

42. Ibid. p.V-9.

43. J. Verrett, 'The Effect of 2,4-D, 2,4,5-T and Their Contaminants on the Developing Chicken Embryo'. Paper presented to the Minnesota Legislature, 1976, Division of Toxicology, Bureau of Foods, Food and Drug Administration, Washington D.C. For a summary of this paper, see J. Warnock and J. Lewis, *op.cit.* 1978, p.13 (addendum). In 1975, the US

Department of Health, Education and Welfare also reported that purified samples of 2,4,5-T were teratogenic – a finding that J. Warnock and J. Lewis described as 'finally putting to rest the notion that the dioxin contaminants are responsible for the teratogenic effects of the phenoxy herbicides'. (J. Warnock and J. Lewis, *op.cit.* 1978, p.11-11.) See also: US Department of Health, Education and Welfare, *2,4,5-T Teratology Study*, Draft Report, Jefferson, Ark. NCTR Branch, 1975.

44. J. Lewis, personal communication, 1979.

45. In 1963, the US Food and Drugs Administration conducted a study on the effects of 2,4,-D on dogs and rats. The study was not made public until 1971. In 1976, according to J. Warnock and J. Lewis, 'the US Environmental Protection Agency cited (those studies) as "sufficient" to satisfy the "chronic" safety testing requirements for re-registration'. Subsequently, Dr Melvin Reuber, a renowned expert in the field, reanalysed the study and concluded: '2,4,-Dichlorophenoxyacetic acid is carcinogenic in rats.' The study was less conclusive about the effects of the herbicide on dogs. See: J. Warnock and J. Lewis, *op.cit.* 1978, p.111-13. In 1978, Richard L. Reising of the Special Pesticide Reviews Division wrote to Gil Zemansky of Friends of the Earth (Seattle) and said: 'The (EPA's) Cancer Assessment Group through an informal review found positive evidence that 2,4,-D is carcinogenic.' J. Warnock and J. Lewis released Reising's letter to the Canadian media: immediately there was near panic in Washington. The 'informal' study to which the letter referred was that by Melvin Reuber. EPA headquarters, however, were at pains to point out that Reuber's reanalysis had not been undertaken officially: 'Officially, the Cancer Assessment Group did not conduct an "informal review" of 2,4-D, therefore we have nothing official to support the claim made in (Reising's) letter.' Even though the matter would best have been resolved through new studies, the EPA made it clear that it was not prepared to initiate such an undertaking.

46. J. Warnock and J. Lewis, *op.cit.* 1978, p.IV-3.

47. 'Herbicide Linked to Miscarriages in West Montana', *New York Herald Tribune*, 11.2.78.

48. J. Warnock and J. Lewis, *op.cit.* 1978, p.IV-8.

49. J. Crossland, 'Dioxin – The Lingering Controversy', *The Ecologist*, Vol. 10, No.3, March 1980, p.80.

50. Jeffery Smith, 'EPA Halts Most Uses of Herbicide 2,4,5-T', *Science*, 16.3.79, p.1090.

51. P. Keisling, 'The Spraying of Oregon, Parts I-IV', *Williamette Weekly*, November-December 1979.

52. J. Cook and C. Kaufman, *Portrait of a Poison: The 2,4,5-T Story*, Pluto, London, 1982, p.89.

53. The episode described here is based upon a sworn statement by Geoffrey Hellier, November 1979. See also: J. Cook and C. Kaufman, *op.cit.* 1982.

54. G. Hellier, Statutory Declaration, Taunton, 5.11.79, p.2.

55. Ibid. p.3. Cook and Kaufman (*op.cit.* 1982, p.39) report: 'Publicity given to what happened ruined (Hellier) as he has been unable to sell any stock because of fear of a health risk. A tenant farmer, he is now penniless and faces eviction.'

56. Report from the Veterinary Investigation Centre, Bristol, 19.6.78.

57. G. Hellier, Sworn Statement, 6.9.78.

58. Advisory Committee on Pesticides, *Further Review of the Safety for Use in the UK of the Herbicide 2,4,5-T.* HMSO, London, 1980, pp.35-38.

59. E. Sigmund, *Rage Against the Dying*, Pluto, London, 1980.

60. I am extremely grateful to Tony Charles and the Ecology Party for supplying details of British cases of phenoxy herbicide poisoning.

61. J. Lewis, 'Spray That Could be Causing Miscarriages', *Guardian,* 18.6.79.

62. Ibid.

63. *Econews*, 'Danger 2,4,5-T', December 1979: Cook and Kaufman, *op.cit.* 1982, p.39.

64. *Econews, op.cit.* 1979: Cook and Kaufman, *op.cit.* 1982, p.38-39.

65. Advisory Committee on Pesticides, *op.cit.* 1980, p.35.

66. B. Young: Statement, 9 January 1980, Ecology Party Dossier on 2,4,5-T.

67. E. Smail, 'Meaningless Answer', letter *Sussex Express,* October 1979.

68. Advisory Committee on Pesticides, *op.cit.* 1980, p.10.

69. Advisory Committee on Pesticides, *op.cit.* 1979, p.8.

70. Ibid. p.7.

71. Ibid. p.6.

72. E. Goldsmith, *op.cit.* 1980, p.103: Royal Commission on Environmental Pollution, Seventh Report, 1979, HMSO, London, p.77. The Royal Commission considered it anomalous that 'at a time when there is concern about the hazards posed by toxic chemicals in the environment and when statutory controls designed to ensure adequate testing of new chemicals have been introduced or are envisaged in most industrial countries, the control of pesticides (in the UK) should continue on a non-statutory basis'.

73. See E. Goldsmith, *op.cit.* 1980 for an excellent account of British legislation on pesticide and the failure of existing controls.

74. Advisory Committee on Pesticides, *op.cit.* 1979, p.9.

75. E. Goldsmith, *op.cit.* 1980, p.109.

76. B. Price, 'Pesticides: Handle with Care', *Guardian*, 18.10.80.

77. Quoted in E. Goldsmith, *op.cit.* 1980, pp.107-108.

78. Reply of Jerry Wigan for the Ministry of Agriculture, Fisheries and Food in answer to parliamentary questions, 18 December 1979. Quoted in press release of Dr Roger Thomas MP, 'A Statement on the Usage in the UK of 2,4,5-T', 9 June 1980. For an excellent account of how Thomas and his colleagues unearthed the true figure for 2,4,5-T usage in Britain, see Cook and Kaufman, *op.cit.* 1982, pp.27-33.

79. R. Thomas, *op.cit.* 1980, p.2.

80. Ibid. p.5.

81. S. Epstein, *op.cit.* 1979, p.302. Chapter 8 (p.299 ff.), provides one of the best accounts available of attempts by industry to distort or suppress relevant data on pesticide tests.

82. EDF and R. Boyle, *op.cit.* 1980, pp.118-119.

83. Quoted in S. Epstein, *op.cit.* 1979, p.303.

84. EDF and R. Boyle, *op.cit.* 1980, p.134.

85. M. Reuber, Testimony before the Senate Committee on Labour and Public Welfare, *Preclinical and Clinical Testing*, Part 1. Washington D.C., 1975, p.626 ff. (hereafter: Preclinical Testing, 1).

86. Quoted in EDF and R. Boyle, *op.cit.* 1980, p.135.

87. S. Epstein, *op.cit.* 1979, p.279.

88. Ibid. pp.273-281: EDF and Boyle, *op.cit.* 1980, p.135.

89. S. Epstein, *op.cit.* 1979, p.273.

90. *Preclinical Testing* 1, *op.cit.* 1975, p.132.

91. S. Epstein, *op.cit.* 1979, p.278.

92. R. Lightfoot, Testimony before the Subcommittee on Crime of the House Committee of the Judiciary, US House of Representatives, Washington D.C., 1980, pp.3-4.

93. Ibid. p.3.

94. Ibid. pp.3-4.

95. Ibid. p.4.

96. Ibid. p.4.

97. Ibid. p.5.

98. R. Watanuki, 'Mercury and Kepone: Two Killers on Two Continents', *Alternatives*, Winter 1978, p.8. March 1977, p.30.

99. Ibid. p.9: F.S. Sterrett and C.A. Boss, 'Careless Kepone', *Environment,* Vol. 19, No.2, March 1977, p.30.

100. According to Dr R.S. Jackson, a state epidemiologist for Virginia, an inspection of the plant revealed 'massive building, air and ground contamination with kepone . . . a chemical odour strong enough to irritate the eyes . . . and no evidence of personal protection except for hard hats'. See: Congressional Research Service, *Background Material Requested For Use in Consideration of HR 7040*, Washington D.C., 1980, p.22. (Hereafter: CRS).

101. S. Epstein, *op.cit.* 1979, p.309.

102. R. Watanuki, *op.cit.* 1978, p.8.

103. As a result of the National Cancer Institute study, the US National Institute of Occupational Safety and Health determined that kepone was a potential human carcinogen. See: CRS, *op.cit.* 1980, p.23: US Department of Health, Education and Welfare, National Institutes of Health, National Cancer Institute, *Carcinogenesis Bio-Assay of Technical Grade Clordecone (Kepone)*, Bethseda, 1976.

104. F.S. Sterrett and C.A. Boss, *op.cit.* 1977, p.32.

105. S. Epstein, *op.cit.* 1979, p.264.

106. Ibid. p.269.

107. Ibid, p.260.

108. Ibid. pp.256-259. Epstein gives a detailed account of the controversy over aldrin and dieldrin.

109. Ibid. p.262.

110. Quoted in S. Epstein, *op.cit.* 1979, p.251.

111. Ibid. p.267.

112. R. Van den Bosch, *The Pesticide Conspiracy*, Doubleday, New York, 1978, p.59.

113. Ibid. p.64.

114. E. Goldsmith, 'Pesticides Create Pests', *The Ecologist*, March 1980, p.94. Van den Bosch notes: '[In the late 1950s] the United States used roughly 50 million pounds of insecticides, [whilst] insects destroyed about 7 per cent of US crops: today (1978), under a 600-million-pound insecticide load, (the US) is losing 13 per cent of (its) preharvest yield to rampaging insects'. (Van den Bosch, *op.cit.* 1978, p.28).

115. Van den Bosch, *op.cit.* 1978, p.11. 'Many insects also have incredible reproductive abilities which are realised through fantastic egg-laying capacities or by the rapid turnover of generations. The champion egg layer is probably the termite, which pumps out about 150 million eggs during her fecund life span. The quick-cycle artists are such creatures as the aphids, which under optimum conditions can turn over a generation a week. The numbers that the insectan birth machines grind out are truly mind-boggling. For example, a locust swarm may cover six hundred square miles and contain more than a trillion insects.'

116. Anil Agarwal, 'Pesticide Resistance on the Increase, says UNEP', *Nature*, Vol. 279, 24.5.79, p.280: 'In 1965, the Food and Agricultural Organisation listed 182 resistant strains of arthropod pests: in 1968, it listed 228 resistant species; and now its latest survey of 1977 lists 364 species.'

117. R. Van den Bosch, *op.cit.* 1978, pp.23-25.

118. Rachel Carson, *Silent Spring*, Houghton Mifflin, New York, 1962.

119. Frank Graham Jnr. *Since Silent Spring*, Hamish Hamilton, London, 1977.

120. Ibid.

121. J. McCaul, 'Questions For an Old Friend', *Environment*, July 1971, p.9.

122. CBNS Notes 2 (5):3, 1969, report on address by Dr. Goran Lofroth, Centre for Biology of Natural Systems, Washington University, St Louis, Missouri.

123. E. Goldsmith, *op.cit.* 1980, p.106.

124. Ibid. p.106.

125. David Weir and Mark Shapiro, *Circle of Poison: Pesticides and People in a Hungry World,* Institute for Food and Development Policy, San Francisco, 1981, p.3.

126. US General Accounting Office, *Better Regulation of Pesticide Exports and Pesticide Residues in Imported Food is Essential*, Report No. CED 79-43, 1979, pp.iii,39.

127. Weir and Shapiro, *op.cit.* 1981, p.21.

128. US GAO, *op.cit.* 1979.

129. Weir and Shapiro, *op.cit.* 1981, pp.29-30.

130. Ibid., update sheet.

131. Anil Agarwal, 'Pesticide Poisoning – Another Third World Disease,' *New Scientist* 21.10.78, p.917: Weir and Shapiro, *op.cit.* 1978, p.11.

132. R. Van den Bosch, *op.cit.* p.30.

Chapter 6: Acid Rain: The Poison from the Skies

1. John Roberts, Minister of the Environment in Canada, quoted in 'The Silent Scourge', Russ Hoyle, *Time Magazine*, 8.11.1982.

2. Renaud Vie le Sage, 'Les Pluies Acides: un Holocauste Ecologique', *La Researche*, No.131, March 1982, p.394.

3. Jacques-Yves Cousteau *et al*, *The Cousteau Almanac*, Columbus B Books, 1981, p.188.

4. Ellis B. Cowling, 'Acid Precipitation in Historical Perspective', *Environmental Science and Technology*, Vol. 16, No.2, 1982, p.110A ff.

5. Ibid. p.111A.

6. R.A. Smith, *Air and Rain: The Beginnings of a Chemical Climatology*, Longmans/Green, London, 1872.

7. Ellis B. Cowling, *op.cit.* 1982.

8. Russ Hoyle, *op.cit.* 8.11.82, p.39.

9. Quoted in Erik Eckholm, *Down to Earth*, Pluto, 1982, p.116.

10. Erik Eckholm, *op.cit.* 1982, p.119.

11. M. Holgate *et al*, *The World Environment*, Tycooly International, Dublic, 1982, p.23.

12. J.-Y. Cousteau, *op.cit.* 1981, p.188.

13. Russ Hoyle, *op.cit.* 1982, p.40.

14. E. Eckholm, *op.cit.* 1982, p.121.

15. Geoffrey Lean, 'The Awful Secret of that Lake that Died'. *Observer*, 19.9.82.

16. Ellis B. Cowling, *op.cit.* 1982, p.110A.

17. Tony Samstag, 'Last Stop on the Pollution Pipeline', *The Times*, 9.9.82.

18. Fred Pearce, 'The Menace of Acid Rain', *New Scientist*, 12.8.82, p.423.

19. Ibid. p.240.

20. Ibid. p.420.

21. J.-Y. Cousteau, *op.cit.* 1981, p.187.

22. 'A Killing Rain', Horizon, BBC Television, 1982, Transcript, pp.33 and 44.

23. Quoted in Fred Pearce, 'The Menace of Acid Rain', *New Scientist*, 12.8.82, p.422.

24. Fred Pearce, 'Warning Cones Hoisted as Acid Rain Clouds Gather', *New Scientist*, 26.8.82, p.828.

25. Fred Pearce, 'It's an Acid Wind That Blows Nobody Any Good', *New Scientist*, 8.7.82, p.80.

26. Ibid.

27. Marek Mayer, 'Britain Slashes Research on Air Pollution', *New Scientist*, 29.4.82, p.271.

28. Tony Samstag, 'Acid Rain Falling Throughout Britain', *The Times,* 20.8.82.

29. Fred Pearce, 'Science and Politics Don't Mix at Acid Rain Debate', *New Scientist*, 1.7.82, p.3.

30. 'A Killing Rain', *op.cit.* 1982.

31. Eliot Marshall, 'Air Pollution Clouds US Canadian/US Relations', *Science*, 17.9.82, pp.1118-1119.

32. Fred Pearce, *op.cit.* 8.7.82.

Chapter 7: Thalidomide and After

1. The *Sunday Times* Insight Team, *Suffer the Children*, Andre Deutsch, London, 1979.

2. Ibid. p.27.

3. Ibid. p.53.

4. Ibid. p.32.

5. Ibid. p.31.

6. Ibid. pp.33-35.

7. Ibid. pp.37.

8. Ibid. p.37.

9. Ibid. pp.38-39.

10. Ibid. pp.60-62.

11. Ibid. p.75.

12. Ibid. p.72.

13. Ibid. p.70.

14. Ibid. pp.87-90.

15. Ibid. pp.99-100.

16. Ibid. p.106.

17. Ibid. p.108.

18. Ibid. p.108.

19. Ibid. p.2.

20. *Preclinical and Clinical Testing by the Pharmaceutical Industry*, 1979, Hearing before the Subcommittee on Health and Scientific Research of the Committee on Labour and Human Resources United States Senate, 96th Congress, Washington D.C., 1979, pp.23-24. (Hereinafter referred to as *Preclinical Testing* IV).

21. Quoted in *Preclinical and Clinical Testing*, Part II. Joint Hearings before the Subcommittee on Health of the Committee on Labour and Public Welfare and the Subcommittee on Administrative Practice and Procedure of the Committee on the Judiciary, US Senate, Washington D.C., 1976, p.157. (Hereinafter referred to as *Preclinical Testing* II).

22. Dr Ian StJames-Roberts 'Cheating in Science', *New Scientist*, 25.11.76.

23. *Preclinical Testing* II, *op.cit.* 1976, p.157.

24. O. Gillie, 'Drug Company Ignored Deformity Risk for Ten Years', *Sunday Times*, 23.4.78.

25. Ibid.

26. Ibid.

27. Ibid.

28. Sidney Wolfe, Testimony before Subcommittee on Crime of the House Judiciary Committee, Washington D.C., 1980, p.62.

29. Ibid. p.62.

30. Ibid. p.64.

31. *Preclinical and Clinical Testing*, Part I. Hearing before the Subcommittee on Health and Scientific Research of the Committee on Labour and Human Resources, US Senate, Washington D.C., 1975, pp.168. (Hereinafter referred to as *Preclinical Testing* I.

32. Ibid. p.169.

33. Ibid. pp.137-139. An earlier inspection team had recommended against prosecution. According to Commissioner Schmidt, it was 'concluded that the management of Lederle had acted properly as soon as it was aware of the alarming finding of bladder carinoma.' The failure of Lederle pathologists to determine that the gross findings were alarming (was described as 'a question of scientific judgement'). (p.138).

34. *Preclinical Testing* IV, *op.cit.* 1979, pp.28-29.

35. Elaine Potter 'Pregnancy Drug Firm Sets Private Eye to "investigate" Expert Witness', *Sunday Times*, 21.9.80.

36. Ibid. (Richardson-Merrel maintained such activities were 'standard practice'.)

37. Gina Bari Kolata, 'Jury Exonerates Bendectin in Mekdeci Case', *Science*, 8.5.81, p.647.

38. *Science*, 31.10.80, p.518.

39. Andrew Veitch, 'Debendox Risk "not proved" Says Report'. *Guardian,* 10.7.81. Mr Barry Hall of the Debendox Action Group, argued that 'the sample is too small. I don't know how you can detect a drug suspected of causing deformities in 5 in 1,000 cases by looking at 620.' (See also: R. Jeffrey Smith 'Studies Support Bendectin Safety Claim', *Science,* 26.6.81, p.1485.

40. Elaine Potter, 'Debendox Hazard Warning – But Not in Britain', *Sunday Times*, 4.7.82. One study, for the German Health Ministry, suggested a link between Debendox and diaphragmatic hernia; the other, a link between Debendox and the development of a heart defect. According

to Potter, a spokesman for DOW Chemicals, (which markets the drug in the USA with Merrells), said the company did not consider 'the (German) findings to be very relevant,' as the researchers had used dosages far above those which would be prescribed for humans. The second study, on monkeys, was performed without using a control group of untreated animals. Both studies were being repeated at the time of writing. For its part, the British Committee on the Safety of Medicines did 'not feel that the studies (provided) scientifically acceptable evidence that the drug (causes) damage'. In 1981, however, the British government had issued the following warning: 'there have been a large number of epidemiological studies of Debendox. Although there have been some reports of congenital malformations associated with its administration in early pregnancy, a causal relationship has not been established. For no medicinal product can a small risk of teratogenic effect (causing deformity to embryos) be excluded with absolute certainty, and so the use of any drug during early pregnancy should be avoided if at all possible.'

41. *Preclinical Testing* I, *op.cit.* 1975, pp.51-52.
42. Ibid. pp.51-52.
43. Ibid. pp.52-53.
44. Ibid. p.55.
45. Ibid. p.56.
46. Ibid. p.57.
47. Ibid. p.57.
48. On Nov. 11th 1981, Searle wrote to New English Library complaining that my handling of this and other incidents involving Searle appeared 'to demonstrate an intentional and malicious disregard for the truth'. With regard to my reporting of the Flagyl episode, the company stated: 'Fact: pages 253-261 of the testimony of the first session of the Joint Hearings demonstrate that embedding tissue in paraffin does not make the tissue unanalyzable. The tissue was analyzed and it was tissue from a male as reported by Searle.' In his evidence before the Committee (ibid. pp.186-197) Dr Buzzard of Searle said: 'Contrary to what Dr Gross implies, embedding does not preclude a test for sex identification. We ran such a test on the block in question last night, after first learning of his purpose yesterday. Our preliminary results indicate that (the) rat in question was, and the tissue still is, from a male. We would welcome others to . . . run tests of their own.' In his rebuttal testimony, Gross replied: 'I do not know whether embedding indeed "does not preclude a test for sex identification" as Dr Buzzard testified. The field of genetics is not my own speciality and what Searle asserts now can only be evaluated by experts in this particular field. My own information at that time (gathered from Dr Sydney Green, the head of the genetics laboratory at the Food and Drugs Administration) was that fresh tissue was the ideal material for chromosome analysis, formalin fixed (wet) tissue is somewhat less suitable for this purpose and paraffin infiltrated tissue least if at all so,' (p.477).

49. *Preclinical Testing* I, *op.cit.* 1975, p.63.

50. Ibid. p.64.

51. Ibid. p.441. Also *Preclinical Testing* II, *op.cit.* 1976, p.64.

52. Ibid. p.66.

53. In the first edition of *Cover-Up*, I mistakenly alleged that Dr George McConnell had shown the faulty table. In fact, it was Dr Weil; Dr *Robert* McConnell is a Searle employee who attended the meeting. I am grateful to Searle for pointing out this error and apologise to Dr G. McConnell. In their letter of 11 November 1981 to New English Library (see reference 48), Searle stated: 'Fact: Pages 235-248 of the record of the first session of the Joint Hearings demonstrate that Dr *Robert* McConnell, a Searle *employee*, did show the meeting participants a table with all tumours reported.' This is true; (p.445-446).

54. *Preclinical and Clinical Testing* II, *op.cit.* 1976, pp.14-15.

55. Ibid. pp.20-23.

56. Ibid. p.76.

57. For example, in their letter of 11 November 1981 (see reference 48), Searle wrote: 'Dr Waisman, a renowned authority in phenylalanine, was a consultant to Searle. Dr Waisman on his own volition began a small pilot study in monkeys involving large doses of aspartame which contains phenylananine. Before Dr Waisman completed his study he died. Searle, based on documents obtained from Dr Waisman's laboratory after his death, submitted a report to the FDA based on those documents. Searle could not then or now answer detailed questions about Dr Waisman's work. Searle did discuss doing a large controlled study with Dr Waisman to determine the effects of large doses of aspartame on monkeys. This study was described as 'of the first priority to Searle'. Because of Dr Waisman's death, this study was ultimately done by other scientists and reported to the FDA.'

58. *Preclinical and Clinical Testing* II, *op.cit.* 1976, p.17-19.

59. Ibid. p.19.

60. David Dickson, 'Aspartame Sugar Substitute: New Court Overruled', *Nature* Vol. 292, 23.7.81, p.283. In February 1980, a 'science court' of three independent scientists had ruled against permission being granted for aspartame to be marketed. The FDA overruled the science court after its Bureau of Foods concluded that 'the sweetener would be safe at the "highest conceivable levels" of consumption.' At the time that the science court made its decision, reports Dickson, 'Searle were sitting on a stockpile of 300,000 lbs of the sweetener with a market value of over £25 million.' Two years of independent auditing had exonerated the company of accusations that its animal studies were invalid. *See also*: R. Jeffrey Smith, 'Aspartame Approved Despite Risks', *Science*, Vol. 213, 28.8.81, pp.986-987.

61. Epstein, *op.cit.* 1979, p.309.

62. *Preclinical and Clinical Testing*, *op.cit.* 1977, p.158 and p.159.

63. S. Epstein, *op.cit.* 1979, p.309.
64. Ibid, p.310.
65. *Preclinical and Clinical Testing* IV, *op.cit.* 1979, pp.40-41.
66. Ibid. p.42.

Chapter 8: Asbestos— The Slow Killer

1. Alan Dalton, *Asbestos: Killer Dust*, British Society for Social Responsibility in Science, London, 1979, p.15.
2. Ibid. p.17.
3. Philip L. Polakoff, Testimony to Subcommittee on Compensation, Health and Safety of House Committee on Education and Labour, US House of Representatives, Washington D.C., 1978, p.132.
4. H.M. Murray, in *Report of the Departmental Committee on Compensation for Industrial Disease* (Minutes of Evidence, Appendices and Index), London, 1907.
5. W.E. Cooke, 'Fibrosis of the Lungs due to the inhalation of Asbestos Dust' *British Journal of Medicine*, II, 26.7.24.
6. E. Merewether and C. Price, *Report on Effects of Asbestos Dust on the Lungs and Dust Suppression in the Asbestos Industry*, HMSO London, 1930: B. Castleman, Statement before the Subcommittee on Crime of the House Judiciary Committee, US House of Representatives, Washington D.C., 1979, p.7.
7. E. Merewether, 'The Occurrence of Pulmonary Fibrosis and Other Pulmonary Affections in Asbestos Workers'. *Journal of Industrial Hygiene*, 12, 1930, pp.198-222, 239-257.
8. S. Epstein, *The Politics of Cancer*, Doubleday/Anchor, New York, 1979, p.81: B. Castleman, *op.cit.* 1979, pp.8,16.
9. S. Epstein, *op.cit.* 1979, pp.81-82. The death rate was 50 per cent higher than the average white male.
10. K. Carlson, 'Asbestos' Chronological Highlight'. Statement before Subcommittee on Compensation, Health and Safety of the House Committee on Education and Labour, House of Representatives, Washington D.C., 1978, p.52. In 1952, Dr Kenneth Smith, Medical Director of Johns-Manville's New Jersey plant, recommended the use of warning labels. The recommendation was overruled. Castleman (*op.cit.* 1979, p.24) quotes Smith as saying: 'The reasons why the caution labels were not implemented immediately, it was a business decision as far as I could understand. Here was a recommendation, the corporation is in business to make, to provide jobs for people and make money for stock-holders and they had to take into consideration the effects of everything they did and if the application of a caution label identifying a product as hazardous would cut into sales, there would be serious financial implications. And the powers that be had to make some effort to judge the necessity of the label versus the consequences of placing the label on the

product.' (English as in original).

11. R.W. Moss, *The Cancer Syndrome*, Grove Press Inc./New York, 1980, p.242.

12. Ibid. p.242.

13. S. Epstein, *op.cit.* 1979, pp.81-82. The group of workers 'had experienced a death rate 50 per cent greater than the average white male. Among these 'excess' deaths, lung cancer by far exceeded the expected experience of such a group of men by a factor of seven.

14. R. Moss, *op.cit.* 1980, p.243.

15. S. Epstein, *op.cit.* 1979, p.90.

16. B. Castleman, *op.cit.* 1979, p.8.

17. Ibid. p.9.

18. Letter from Hobart to Brown, December 15th, 1934.

19. Letter from Brown to Lanza, December 21st, 1934.

20. B. Castleman, *op.cit.* 1979, p.9.

21. Minutes of Board Meeting, Johns-Manville, 24.4.33.

22. Letter from *Asbestos* to Brown, October 1st 1935.

23. Letter from Simpson to Brown, October 1st 1935.

24. Letter from Brown to Simpson, October 3rd 1935.

25. Letter from Simpson to Blagden, November 10th 1936.

26. B. Castleman, *op.cit.* 1979, p.11.

27. Ibid. p.11.

28. S. Epstein, *op.cit.* 1979, p.93.

29. B. Castleman, *op.cit.* 1979, p.26.

30. Ibid. p.19.

31. Ibid. p.19.

32. Ibid. p.20.

33. Ibid. p.23.

34. Interview with Mancuso, Pittsburg, 1980. Mancuso wrote at the time: 'Internally, within the company, the question has to be raised as to why medical problems, particularly relating to cancer and asbestos were not recognised before. Actually, they were recognised, but the asbestos industry chose to ignore and deny their existence.' (Quoted by B. Castleman, *op.cit.* 1979, p.23).

35. Neville Hodgkinson, 'Asbestos Dangers Threaten a £200 Million Industry', *The Times*, 28.3.77.

36. Barry Castleman and M.J. Vera Vera, 'The Selling of Asbestos', *The Ecologist*, Vol. 11 No.3, 1981, pp. 109-110. 'The international asbestos industry's own view of its responsibility to label its products as potentially lethal was recently revealed by the disclosure of an internal memorandum of the Asbestos International Association dated July 7 1978. The industry members generally agreed that it would be best to get by with as little warning labelling as their various markets would bear: "Most participants were in favour of an action in various stages, the switching over from one stage to a further less favourable one, depending on outside pressure." The

British asbestos industry's approach to the labelling problem was regarded by many observers as worthy of imitation. This is because the British firms have been able to get their government off their backs with a warning label that reads, "Take care with asbestos." The memorandum goes on to note: "Many of the participants were of the opinion that it was advisable to adopt the UK label as such *if the use of a label was unavoidable. Rediscussing the wording could bring along the risk of having to include the word "cancer" in it.* The fact that this label had been found satisfactory to the UK authorities was also seen as a good argument for avoiding the EEC (European Economic Community) to press for a less favourable one (such as the skull-and-crossbones used for "toxic substances").' (Emphasis added.) The industry appeared unanimous, however, in the view that the best warning label is none at all. *"In those countries where it was felt still too early to start voluntary labelling, in fear of a negative influence on sales,* steps should be taken in order to prepare commercial people for the idea, making clear that in the absence of an industry's initiative we could run the risk of being imposed the "skull-and-crossbones" symbol for our products. It should also be pointed out to them that the fact to agree on a kind of label did not imply the agreement of starting to use it right now.' (Emphasis added.)

37. A. Dalton, *op.cit.* 1979, p.121.

38. Ibid. p.122.

39. S. Epstein, *op.cit.* 1979, pp.83-84.

40. Ibid. p.87. The British asbestos industry argued that even to reduce the level to twice the proposed NIOSH standard (i.e. 0.2 fibres per cubic centimetre) would mean the wholesale closure of British asbestos factories and the loss of 20,000 jobs. See, Neville, Hodgkinson, *op.cit.* 1977.

41. 'Asbestos limit cut', *Guardian*, 25.8.82.

42. Angela Singer, 'More Time to Do Nothing'. *Guardian*, 6.8.82. 'The one fibre standard . . . is an arbitrary level. It cannot be accurately measured in the factory. The Health and Safety Executive admits an error factor in the counting of fibres of at least 50 per cent.'

43. David Nicholson-Lord, 'Asbestos Dust Levels to be Cut', *The Times*, 25.8.82. According to the Health and Safety Commission nine-tenths of the asbestos industry work to the 1 fibre standard. See also ref. 41: 'The proposed reduction was criticised by the General and Municipal Workers Union, which (had) been pressing for a reduction to 0.5 fibres per cubic centimetre. The Union's national officer, Mr Frank Earl said: 'The proposed one fibre limit would still result in the deaths of one in ten workers and illness to countless more." '

44. Angela Singer, *Guardian*, 11.9.79.

45. *Twenty Sensible Questions You Asked About Asbestos,* Advertisement sponsored by the Asbestos Information Committee, *The Times*, 1.7.76.

46. A. Dalton, *op.cit.* 1979, pp.29-34. See also, Subcommittee on Compensation, Health and Safety of the House Committee on Education and

Labour, *Asbestos Related Occupational Disease*, House of Representatives, Washington D.C., 1978, pp.13, 149, 158.

47. Benjamin Suta, Statement before Subcommittee on Compensation, Health and Safety of the House Committee on Education and Labour, *Asbestos Related Occupational Disease*, House of Representatives, Washington D.C., 1978, pp.9-16.

48. Quoted in E. Goldsmith, 'Can We Control Pollution?' *The Ecologist*, Vol. 9, No.8, 1979.

49. A. Dalton, *op. cit.* 1979, p.7. In 1982, Dr Selikoff predicted that one American would be killed 'every 50 minutes between now and the end of the century' as a result of exposure to asbestos. (See: 'Alice, A Fight for Life', Full Transcript, Yorkshire Television, 1982, p.27).

50. S. Solomon, 'The Asbestos Fall-Out at Johns-Manville' *Fortune*, 7.5.79, pp.196-206.

51. Barnaby J. Feder, 'Asbestos Injury Suits Mount, With Serious Impact', *New York Times*, 3.7.81. Under Chapter 11 of the US Bankruptcy Act, the company can still trade. Indeed after it declared itself bankrupt, JM placed full page advertisements in leading newspapers assuring readers: 'Nothing is wrong with our business.' (See J. Erlichman and H. Jackson 'Asbestos Firms Close Ranks on Claim', *Guardian*, 28.8.82.)

52. Nicholas Hirst, 'Manville Bankruptcy Move After Lawsuits', *The Times*, 27.8.82.

53. Philip Robinson, 'World Insurers Pay Out £58,000 Million For Asbestosis', *The Times*, 8.8.82.

54. Yorkshire TV, 'Alice, a Fight for Life,' Full Transcript, 2.8.82, p.59.

55. 'Asbestos Denial', *Guardian*, 23.7.82. See also, Andrew Veitch, 'Health and Safety Chief Denies Asbestos Claim', *Guardian*, 4.9.82. According to Bill Simpson, Chairman of the inquiry, Morris' findings were 'passed informally' to Dr Ken Duncan, chairman of the inquiry's medical working group and his paper was 'subsequently seen by all the members of the medical working group.' Andrew Veitch reports, however, that Dr Martin Gardner, an epidemiologist at Southampton University who prepared the scientific evidence for the inquiry could not recall seeing the document. 'I have no recollection of seeing it but I cannot be absolutely sure. I have no memory of any document from Dr Morris nor do we have any such paper on our files.'

56. Angela Singer, 'Asbestosis Firm Back-pedals on Cancer Statistics', *Guardian*, 18.8.82.

57. Ibid.

58. 'T + N Shares Cut Back to 25p' *The Times*, 4.9.82.

59. B. Castleman, 'The Export of Hazardous Factories to Developing Nations', *International Journal of Health Services*, Vol. 9, No.4, 1979, p.576.

60. Ibid. p.576. See also: G. Yoakum, 'Workers Inhale Deadly Asbestos', *Arizona Daily Star*, 27.3.77.

61. B. Bastleman, *op.cit.* 1979, p.576. See also G. Yoakum, 'Asbestos Pressure Dwindles', *Arizona Daily Star*, 30.5.77.

62. B. Castleman and M.J. Vera Vera, 'The Selling of Asbestos', *The Ecologist*, Vol. 11, No.3, 1981, p.115.

63. Letter, *New Scientist*, 2.4.81, p.45. N. Venkataraman argues: 'every statement (Castleman) makes about the plant is untrue . . . over the past six years the Bombay factory inspectorate has been so impressed by Hindustan Ferodo's dust control that it has arranged for representatives from local cotton textile mills to visit the plant to learn from the methods we employ.'

64. Martin Bailey, 'Shock Report on UK Asbestos Firm', *Observer*, 15.8.82. The report had been presented at the 5th International Symposium on Inhaled Particles in Cardiff, September 1980, but had not been published by the time the *Observer* article appeared. Although it was never alleged that it had done so, T + N denied having suppressed the report ('Asbestos Report', *Letter* from H. Hardie), *Observer*, 22.8.82.

65. M. Bailey, *op.cit.* 15.8.82.

66. M. Hardie, Letter, *Observer*, 22.8.82.

Chapter 9: Lead: The Poison in our Petrol

1. D. Bryce-Smith and R. Stephens, *Lead or Health*? Conservation Society, London, 1980. Dr Waldron, a member of the controversial Lawther Committee, points out: 'On an industrial scale, lead poisoning is still the most common form of industrial pollution.' (H. Waldron, 'Lead Damages Haem-enzymes', *Doctor*, 18.6.81, p.28.

2. Quoted in J. Matthews, 'The Lead Battle Enters the Courts', *New Scientist*, 13.7.78, p.119.

3. J. Matthews, *op.cit.* A. Mackie et al, *Archives of Environmental Health,* no.32, p.178.

4. J. Matthews, *op.cit.* p.118. Stephens took children to mean those under 13 years of age.

5. J. Matthews, *op.cit.* p.119. The official report of the committee assured the public that 'the studies have not shown any cause for special concern about lead pollution from such concentrations of traffic as around Gravelly Hill (Spaghetti Junction)'.

6. Undoubtedly Stephens' mistake was to issue a statement voicing his own misgivings about the study at press conferences held by the DOE to launch the official report. (See J. Matthews, *op.cit.*)

7. Des Wilson, 'Petrol: Must our Children Still be Poisoned?' *The Times*, 8.2.82: J. Matthews, 'The Case Against Lead in Petrol' *New Scientist,* 11.8.77, p.348.

8. 'Lead in Petrol: Your Questions Answered', Conservation Society, October 1973, p.5.

9. Anthony Tucker, *The Toxic Metals*, Pan/Ballantine, London, 1972.

10. Ibid. p.107.

11. Ibid. p.107.
12. Ibid. p.107.
13. A.A. Moncrieff *et al, Archives of Disease in Childhood*, 39, 1964, p.1: D. Bryce-Smith *et al*, 'Mental Health Effects of Lead on Children', *Ambio*, Vol. 7, Nos.5-6, 1978, pp.193-194.
14. D. Bryce-Smith *et al, op.cit.* 1978, pp.193-194.
15. Ibid. pp.193-194.
16. A. Tucker, *op.cit.* 1972, p.102.
17. D. Bryce-Smith *et al, op.cit.* 1978, p.194: A.A. Moncrieff *et al, British Medical Journal*, Vol. 2, 1967, p.480.
18. A. Tucker, *op.cit.* 1972, p.102: N. Gordon *et al, British Medical Journal*, Vol. 2, 1967, p.480.
19. D. Bryce-Smith *et al, op.cit.* 1978, p.194: *Lead Pollution in Birmingham,* HMSO, London, May 1978.
20. R.O. Pihl and M. Parkes, 'Hair Element Content in Learning Disabled Children', *Science* No.198, 1977, p.204: J. Matthews, *op.cit.* 13.7.1978, p.119: N. Kollerstrom, *Lead on the Brain, Wildwood, London,* 1982, p.36.
21. N. Kollerstrom, *op.cit.* 1982, p.38: D. Bryce-Smith *et al, op.cit.* 1978, p.202: G. Winneke *et al*, 'Correlation Between Tooth Lead Levels and Measures of Mental Function in Children', *Medizinches Institut fur Lufthygiene und Silikosforschung an der Universitat,* Dusseldorf.
22. D. Bryce-Smith, *op.cit.* 1978, p.202.
23. N. Kollerstrom, *op.cit.* 1982, p.39: D. Bryce-Smith and R. Stephens, *op.cit.* 1980, p.71.
24. N. Kollerstrom, *op.cit.* 1982, p.39.
25. Ibid. p.97: D. Bryce-Smith and R. Stephens, *op.cit.* 1980, p.71. Commenting on this suggestion, in 1978, La Porte and Talbott remark, 'one wonders whether current limits of lead in the environment are disrupting the development of the extremely complex processes of human thought, such as inferences, metaphors, mathematics, language or logic'. (La Porte and Talbott, *Archives of Environmental Health*, 37, 1978, p.236). See also: G. Winneke *et al, Archives of Toxicology*, 37, (1977), p.248.
26. H. Needleman et al, *New England Journal of Medicine,* 1979, p.689.
27. Ibid. See also N. Kollerstrom, *op.cit.* 1982, p.40: D. Bryce-Smith and R. Stephens, *op.cit.* 1980, p.41.
28. D. Bryce-Smith and R. Stephens, *op.cit.* 1980, p.45.
29. Des Wilson, 'Lead: A Clear Cut Issue?' *The Ecologist*, Vol. 12, No.3. (1982) p.121. In his book, *Lead on the Brain, op.cit.* 1982, p.45, Nick Kollerstrom notes, 'a net displacement downwards on the IQ curve by a mere 5 points would result in a more than 100 per cent increase in children classified as mentally retarded, that is, with an IQ under 70. This follows from the shape of the IQ distribution curve. From 1950 to 1976, institutionalized educational subnormality actually increased more than three times. Other investigations have conclusively shown raised body lead in mentally

subnormal groups of children both in the UK and abroad.'

30. N. Kollerstrom, *op.cit.* 1982, p.40: D. Bryce-Smith and R. Stephens, *op.cit.* 1980, p.41.

31. N. Kollerstrom, *op.cit.* 1982, p.40.

32. Ibid. p.44: V. Garnys *et al*, *Lead Burden of Sydney Schoolchildren,* University of New South Wales, 1979.

33. Quoted in N. Kollerstrom, *op.cit.* 1982, p.44.

34. Ibid. p.44.

35. *Lead and Health*, HMSO, 1980, para.208.

36. N. Kollerstrom, *op.cit.* 1982, pp.50-51.

37. *Lead and Health*, *op.cit.* 1980, para.155.

38. N. Kollerstrom, *op.cit.* 1982, p.36.

39. D. Bryce-Smith and R. Stephens, *op.cit.* 1980, p.43.

40. Ibid. p.42.

41. Ibid. p.43.

42. M. Rutter, Devel. Med. Child. Neurol., 1980, 22, Supplement. No.42,1.

43. In his review, Rutter wrote: 'There are a number of important questions and reservations about the study and the inferences to be drawn from it, but none of these are sufficient to invalidate the findings.' *Lead and Health* on the other hand, reported: 'There are a number of reservations about these studies and the inferences to be drawn from them, which in our view weakens their conclusions.' (para.159).

44. N. Kollerstrom, *op.cit.* 1982, p.51.

45. D. Bryce-Smith and R. Stephens, *op.cit.* 1980, p.43.

46. O.J. David, private communication to D. Bryce-Smith, 21.5.1980.

47. N. Kollerstrom, *op.cit.* 1982, p.36.

48. Ibid. p.35.

49. Ibid. p.35.

50. Ibid. p.35.

51. D. Bryce-Smith and R. Stephens, *op.cit.* 1980, p.97.

52. Ibid. p.33. The controversy over absorption rates has raged for nearly two decades. Yet, as Anthony Tucker points out, 'it is a curious fact that as the concentrations of lead in the urban air have risen, the absorption rates emanating from experimental work by scientists close to the alkyl industry have steadily declined.' (Tucker, *op.cit.* 1972, p.109). What is known is that studies of those living near Spaghetti Junction found that five months after the interchange opened, the levels of lead in the blood of male adults had risen by 31.5 per cent and in female adults by 36.6. per cent: thirteen months later those figures had risen to 64.7 per cent and 75.7 per cent (J. Matthews, *op.cit.* 11.8.77, p.349). An isotope study conducted in Turin, Italy, concluded that 30 per cent of blood lead came from petrol. Moreover, the 50 per cent reduction in lead in petrol achieved in the USA since 1976 had brought a 36.7 lead reduction in the overall mean blood lead level. (See Des Wilson, *The Ecologist*, *op.cit.* 1982, p.121.). Those figures

would suggest far higher absorption rates than those claimed by Lawther or the lead industry – for a full discussion see D. Bryce-Smith and R. Stephens, *op.cit.* 1980, p.32 ff.

53. *Lead and Health*, HMSO 1980, para.208.
54. G. Holmes, Report to Reading Borough Council Environment Committee Minute No.31, RBC Official Minutes, 13.9.78.
55. D. Bryce-Smith and R. Stephens, *op.cit.* 1980, p.19.
56. Ibid. p.20.
57. C. Patterson, *Sierra Studies Report*, California Institute of Technology, 1975, p.2.
58. D. Bryce-Smith and R. Stephens, *op.cit.* 1980, p.18.
59. N. Kollerstrom, *op.cit.* 1982, p.71.
60. R. Russell-Jones, 'Lead Pollution: Why the Government Must Act Now', *World Medicine*, 7.2.81, p.78.
61. Ibid. p.78: B.E. Davies *et al*, *Journal of Agricultural Sciences*, 93, 1979, p.749.
62. N. Kollerstrom, *op.cit.* 1982, p.72.
63. Ibid. p.72.
64. Ibid. p.73.
65. Ibid. p.73.
66. M.A. Healy, *Lead. The Environment And Health*, Nottinghamshire Environment Advisory Council, 1982, p.5.
67. N. Kollerstrom, *op.cit.* 1982, p.74.
68. Ibid. p.77.
69. Ibid. p.77.
70. Ibid. p.77.
71. Ibid. p.77.
72. Ibid. p.77.
73. Ibid. p.78.
74. Ibid. p.78.
75. *Now!*, January 1980, p.50.
76. W. Yule *et al*, *Developmental Medicine and Child Neurology*, 23, 1981, p.567.
77. W. Yule, letter to *The Times*, 10.10.81.
78. A. Tucker, 'Low Lead Levels Affect Children's IQ, Warns Study', *Guardian*, 30.9.81.
79. Ibid.
80. W. Yule, letter to *The Times*, 10.10.81.
81. N. Kollerstrom, *op.cit.* 1982, p.53.
82. Full text of Lead Risk Letter, *The Times,* 8.2.82.
83. N. Kollerstrom, 'About-turn in the Department of Health', article submitted to *The Ecologist*, 1981.
84. The leak prompted a lively correspondence. Sir Henry wrote however, to deny the inferences that had been drawn from his letter: 'It is erroneous to infer that my advice in any way negated or contradicted that of Profes-

sor Lawther's working party on lead and health. The contrary is the case.'

85. Des Wilson, 'Lead, A Clear Cut Issue', *The Ecologist*, Vol. 12, No.3, 1982, p.122.

86. Quoted in Des Wilson, Ibid. p.122.

87. Eliot Marshall, 'White House Steps Into Lead Fight', *Science*, Vol. 217, 27.8.82, p.807.

88. Peter Gwynne, 'Good and Bad News for the US Environment', *New Scientist*, 2.9.82, p.606.

89. Stephen Budianksy, 'EPA Holds Out Against Lead', *Nature*, 2.9.82.

90. Eliot Marshall, 'The Politics of Lead', *Science*, Vol. 216, 30.4.82, p.496.

91. Ibid.

92. S. Budiansky, *op.cit.* 1982.

93. David Beak, 'New Alert Over Lead in Blood', *Sunday Times*, 4.7.82.

Postscript

1. Quoted in Peter Abbs, *Ethical Imagination or the Nuclear Holocaust: Reflections on Education, War and Peace*, 1982, p.5.

2. Ibid. p.5.

3. W. Gebauer, *The Industry and its Operating Environment*, Agrochemical Conference, Zurich, 1981, p.1.

4. New Watt Appointee Nixes Negativism', *Not Man Apart*, December, 1981, p.3.

5. Duncan Burn, *Nuclear Power and the Energy Crisis*, Macmillan, London, 1979.

6. For a fuller discussion of the extent to which the nuclear industry has become a victim of the fortress mentality, see *The Ecologist*, Vol. 11, No.6, 1981, pp.250-253.

INDEX